39 YEARS

Battling with the Bully

Stanley C. James

Produced by Softwood Books, Suffolk, UK
First Edition

ISBN: 978-1-7384605-0-2

www.softwoodbooks.com

Introduction

Well… finally what you are holding is complete and it's been an arduous and sometimes very upsetting but cathartic experience. What you are about to read is a story of more than three decades of painful, challenging, exhausting struggle, involving abuse and bullying, alcoholism, debt, depression, and anger/frustration, leading to planned suicides and years of stress-related health conditions. Some situations may be hard to believe, but everything here in this book did happen the way I have written it.

The book doesn't hold back. I wrote it to make you think and question what you think, as well as consider how you are as parents and people. A lot of it is to do with how bad childhood experiences affect mental health. In the world I live in, mental health problems are often still a taboo subject. So I have chosen to write this book under a pseudonym. I'm not ashamed of the struggles I've had with my mind's health, but I am not a celebrity and nor do I have their wealth. So, I feel that if I want to continue to earn a living in the area I live in, it's best that people do not know I am the author.

I need to just say, this story is not being told for anyone to feel sorry for me – it's being told to show the way my life unfolded. Coming up to fifty years old as I write this, I am hoping people will read it and ask themselves questions and look at others around them and ask questions to those people too. What I really hope is that it will help someone who may be feeling the way I did and that they may find some answers. I know it seems like a sad story (and a good percentage is sad, I suppose), but I am not sad anymore, so please read on.

CHAPTER 1

Background

My earliest memory would have to be at nearly five years old moving from Deal in Kent (England) to a small town in Suffolk called Bury St. Edmunds. Once we had moved there, my parents were on the housing list for a council house, but in the meantime we lived with my grandmother (on my father's side).

With three generations of an extended family living together, life was sometimes difficult. I have some happy memories of being with my Nanna, but plenty of other less happy ones of that time. Of course, I didn't know it then, but the problems had started long before, with my parents' families.

First my mother. She was one of five children living with her own mother and a stepfather. (He was the biological father of the oldest three children, but – as my mother later found out and eventually told me – her mother had a 'fling' with the local bakery delivery man and she was the result.) My grandmother was a manual worker doing menial tasks for low wages, e.g., cleaning or, as I can remember, making Christmas decorations in her kitchen at home. I used to wonder why it was always Christmas at her house, but without goodies. While she was doing this, my granddad (by marriage only) would be in the sitting room watching TV – a close relationship it was not. When he did work, Granddad (as I called him) spent money on himself, pretending to be something he wasn't. (Once, he bought himself a tuxedo to attend a council meeting, even though he wasn't a councillor and had nothing to do with the council!) He would spend money on himself, keeping it from the family, so home life for my mother was quite poor (monetarily speaking). But I do have to say at this point that my mother always looked upon her stepfather as her Dad and said he had always treated her like his own daughter.

Now my mother couldn't lie if her life depended on it – if she says her stepfather was like a dad to her, then that's how it was. She was brought up poor, with worn out shoes with holes in and coats on the beds to try to stay warm, and as far as I can ascertain, her own mother did the best job she could, being the person that she was.

It seems to me that because of her low intelligence and lack of confidence, she didn't have the thinking power to resolve the problem and instead just stayed with the status quo, however wrong it was. Without meaning to sound mean, that was my grandmother's way. Whereas my granddad was more intelligent, but far from being the intellectual that he thought he was. He was a bit of a Walter Mitty character who told stories of accomplishments that he had achieved, and all were made up (or lies, but 'lies' is such a severe word in these circumstances). He didn't say things to hurt anyone, just to make himself feel better or more worthy – a dreamer or pretender, but harmless at heart. To be honest, I think most of the stories he genuinely believed himself. They say that if you can fool yourself, you can fool anyone.

I can remember cycling round to his house on a sunny Sunday morning and discussing an idea I had for a new go-kart, and he seemed really interested. Then he was showing me his latest fish in his aquariums and the pond in the garden. Even at the age of seven or eight, I would think, *How come Granddad has all these fish tanks?* He had two large aquariums in the sitting room (or *his* room as it should have been known and probably was really), plus upstairs in the small spare room there were fish tanks everywhere. They seemed to me to go from the floor to the ceiling down both side walls. I did think then, *How can they afford this?* because I never knew my granddad to work. But I also did realise that my grandmother didn't have a lot either and seemed to be always working in the kitchen making those decorations, always with a cigarette in her mouth. Where the smoke had gone past her face, it would stain all the front of her hair. The whole kitchen was covered in an orangey film, which I later found out to be nicotine, as was the ginger fringe that my grandmother sported. I can still recall that very distinct smell of all that nicotine. What is strange though is that if I went round to their house, my grandmother always would get me a piece of cake and I cannot remember it tasting of smoke or nicotine, whereas later in my life, my ex-father-in-law used to smoke in their kitchen and everything food-wise would have a horrible musty sort of taste.

So, to sum up my mother's parents and her general life, it was a fairly poor childhood but with some love obviously shown from her stepdad that she remembers fondly, and she did have a very strong bond between herself and her mother. Maybe, because she never knew her biological father at all, she kept extremely close to her mother and always felt like the odd one out in the family, and I suppose she was. Not knowing anything about her father apart from his occupation doesn't help when you are trying to make sense of who you are and what you are all about when you only have half the story/background. (That applies to both her and me!)

The best way to describe my mother is that she was always very shy. As a young woman, I would say she was not only shy but very introverted, not outgoing at all. She was and is a lot happier staying around people she knew very well, and she is still that way. She's not and never has been a drinker, nor has she ever smoked. Despite her mother's habit and the fact that all her siblings smoked, she never has. One thing she has is a very stubborn streak. In fact, I would say it's more like a bloody-mindedness. If she gets angered with you, she will just stop speaking to you, which in itself can be very frustrating when she has not even told you what the problem was in the first place. This sort of behaviour, like I say, could be genetic and come from her real father, but since her stepfather would do the same sort of thing, it could be a behavioural trait that she picked up as a little girl.

So we have a shy, introverted person, low in self-belief/confidence (and these are not the same things – you can have either or both), with a very stubborn streak, in a childish way for an adult.

***

My father was born in 1947, the second eldest of five sons of a Welsh soldier and an English woman (known to me as Nanna) in Bury St. Edmunds, Suffolk, England. After the last son was born, they moved to Wales back to my grandfather's home town. (I must say at this point, I only ever met this man twice in my life and that was enough.) When they moved to Wales and my grandfather was back amongst 'his own', his behaviour started to decline. When he lived in Bury St. Edmunds, they lived with my Nanna's parents (my great-grandparents, who, incidentally, I remember very well, especially 'Great Nanna' as I knew her.) In those days, it was not uncommon for a young couple starting out to live with the in-laws, but obviously living with them meant my grandfather had to be on his best behaviour, so once he was out of that environment and among his own friends and family, his behaviour changed.

Now, he was (and I can't take this off him) a seriously hard worker. Very soon after moving back, he had full employment at the local metal works, which was ten miles from the town of Monmouth where they lived, and my grandad would bike this journey in all weathers, then work a ten- to twelve-hour shift throwing sheets of hot metal around and bike back to Monmouth, six days a week.

Unfortunately, my grandfather was also an alcoholic and would not be able to get back home from work without going to the pub, where he would stay until he had either run out of money and/or nobody would buy him a drink, or he passed out, whichever came soonest. Then, if still standing but without money, he would attempt to cycle back home to sleep it off, so on a Friday when he got paid, instead of going straight home – yes, you guessed it – he would go straight to the pub and drink and drink. But fortunately he would always, with a full pocket, run out of puff (drinking-wise) before running out of money. So when he would eventually get home, he still had what was left of his wages and would reluctantly give my Nanna her housekeeping money, which she would then have to hide, because (again, you guessed it) he would take it back in the middle of the week when he had run out of money for drink. Some weeks she didn't get any housekeeping money at all and was (with five sons) forced to beg, steal, and borrow from whatever sources she could, just to put food on the table.

The whole annoying bit of this sorrowful situation was that being a steelworker in those days paid extremely well. Back in the early sixties, most local workers without any trade or skill would be earning around £5-£6 per week, whereas my grandfather earned double that. The fact that he did not spend it on the family really did have an effect, especially on my Nanna who had to beg and grovel to get him to pay any of the bills. Even if he said he had paid, most of the time he was lying, and then they would be constantly chased by the council or bailiffs wanting payment. My Nanna told me once, my grandfather came home one day with a new television so everyone in their street could see him. He said he had bought it outright, which of course was a lie – they only had it for two weeks when a man came round and repossessed it. This scenario also happened with a bicycle he claimed he had bought for my father, only for the same thing to happen a few weeks later.

For my grandmother, this was a very hard life due to this waster she was married to. (I'm not using this terminology aggressively, but literally – a character like him was just wasting everything.) She obviously loved him, or at least in the beginning. I suppose in those days, you 'made your bed so you had to lie on it', and people did stick with it, even in misery, no matter what. It didn't help when society looked upon divorced people (especially women) distastefully. When my grandfather would come home from the pub blind drunk, he would be very aggressive toward my Nanna, and if any of the boys tried to protect her, he would start on them rather than her. Only the two eldest sons would stand up to him initially. On a number of occasions, my Nanna would take a beating at his hands, and without any remorse he would get up the next day and go off to work, saying (if she challenged him) that it was her fault. (What a piece of work).

As I've already said about my grandfather, on the good side, he was a hard worker (in the early years at least). The other thing he could be commended for was the fact that he wasn't a philanderer (womanizer). His sister told us a story about him during the war. (I have to assess each person I got information from because, especially on my father's side, they were quite accomplished liars. But this little Welsh sister of his was a stoical woman with values and principles. In fact, it was quite unbelievable that she and my grandfather were even related. And *she* definitely wasn't a liar.)

My grandfather and his brother were in France, constantly getting bombed by the Germans for a number of months at a time when they found themselves suddenly together (they were in different regiments due to different ages and abilities), both in the same camp. My granddad discovered that his brother was in fact seeing a lady on what seemed to be a regular basis. At this point, my grandfather took this situation up with him and they ended up fighting about it (literally, with fists). You see, my grandfather, although a drunk, wife beater, and selfish beyond belief, disagreed with philandering and did not accept any excuses for what was, in his opinion, very wrong behaviour. I must say, this is one thing I agree with and have had that opinion/ value right to this day. After their altercation, he asked for a further posting to be away from his brother, who he was holding in contempt for his behaviour.

As a little boy, looking up to this tall, large man, my grandfather's brother, I thought he was nice. In fact, I can remember, after a weekend in Wales with these people, I'd wished that *he* was my granddad because he seemed everything you would imagine a granddad to be to a little boy – tall, strong, caring, family-orientated, with his own home and car – a proper granddad. I only met this man twice, but I felt closer to him than to his brother; he had a warmth to him. I am not condoning his wartime behaviour at all, but he said he would never have dreamed of it had he not been in the middle of a war. When he was in the field with bombs dropping all around him, he literally didn't know if he was going to be alive in the morning.

So with this situation, he thought he would (as they say) fill his boots. But quickly, he found that it wasn't sex that he was looking for – what he actually wanted was a companion, a confidante, someone who he could feel very close to, someone like his wife. But he couldn't have her with him as she was hundreds of miles away in England and he was all alone, apart from a few hundred soldiers – hardly the same, hey? I still do not condone adultery, but I can understand his perspective, and who knows what any of us would do in that scenario. But his brother – my grandfather – was not of this opinion or understanding. (Having said all that, I would like to think that I would not, for want of a better word, betray my wife if I was in the same situation.)

I can see why my grandfather could lack-understanding of his brother's behaviour, because, you see, he already had an extra love with him permanently all day and all night, something he could always turn to. And what was his greater love? Simple –

alcohol! You see, my grandfather, when not soldiering, would be drinking, and that love/obsession/addiction can take such a priority over other feelings and emotions that anyone in the grip of it can stand on their high horse and condemn others for what they see as inappropriate behaviour. My grandfather could be very judgmental to others, like his brother, even to the point of not speaking for the remaining years of the war. But who is misbehaving, really? My grandfather used to beat *his* wife. I personally would call *that* inappropriate behaviour at the highest level (in any relationship, be it two men or two women, the beating of either partner, drunk or otherwise, I totally condemn. It is simply wrong.)

Still on the subject of my grandfather, on one particular occasion, he had returned from the pub and taken his anger out on my Nanna and by all accounts left her in a bad way. She would try to cover her injuries, but on this particular day, she visited her sister-in-law (the stoic Welsh lady) and it came out what had been happening. Her sister-in-law called my Nanna's father back in Suffolk and told him what had been occurring.

My great-grandfather was a tall skinny man, very quiet with his head always in a book and known to be very mean with money. (When we would visit my great-grandparents, my great-grandmother would whisper in my ear as she pushed a fifty pence piece into my hand, "That's for you, don't tell your great-grandad.") I never had him down as a man of action, but in this instance he was. He got a message to my Nanna that he would be coming over to Wales to collect them all and wouldn't take no for an answer. I think my Nanna was actually relieved because she was at the end of her tether. So that's what happened. My great-grandfather picked up my Nanna and the youngest four sons, including my father. They all came back to Bury St. Edmunds to live in a three-bedroom terraced house with my great-grandparents. It was very cramped with all seven of them, but it was better than what they'd had to endure. I should mention that although my Nanna was in some ways glad to be out of the situation that she was in (i.e., a violent, turbulent, and dysfunctional marriage), she would sometimes speak of him fondly, but the story nearly always ended in misery.

So, my father's father was a drunk who also had a pretentious streak in him (wanting people in the street he lived in to see the television so they would think, *Ooh, look what the Davies family have got!*) He was also a very arrogant man who wouldn't be told anything. Add that to the selfishness and he really was a bad catch for my Nanna.

I don't want to describe my father yet because I really didn't know who or what he was until many years later when I could look back and had a lot more facts from others. I think it would be better to liken his characteristics to that of his father and mother as we take this journey through the up and coming years.

CHAPTER 2

Early Memories and Primary School

Once we had moved to Bury (short for Bury St. Edmunds), my parents were on the housing list for a council house, but in the meantime, we lived with my grandmother (on my father's side). I called her Nanna (or just Nan), as she preferred that name to Grandmother, which she said was old fashioned and made her feel old – very ironic really because my Nanna, as I remember her back at the age of forty-five, was already sporting a nice blue rinse in her lightly permed hair and a large support girdle holding all unwanted loose bits firmly in place where she felt they should be (or where they once were).

I was always my Nanna's favourite, being the first grandchild. She was desperate to have a granddaughter, really, after not having a daughter herself but instead having five sons. She was to be the one person to constantly show me affection. I can remember living with her and three of the remaining sons all in this three-bedroom council house, all the bedrooms having to be shared. I was in with my Nanna, which at the age of five I really didn't mind – in fact, even at that age, I was more than happy to be with her instead of my parents.

I can remember on one occasion being sent to my room, which, as I've said, was also my Nanna's room, and being told to stay there very early on in the day. I wasn't tired at all, and in those days, I hadn't got a computer to play on or a PlayStation

– my Nanna definitely didn't have a television in the bedroom. Sitting in her bedroom very bored (I also remember how very cold this bedroom was without any central heating), I looked around, much intrigued by the lovely flowered wallpaper. I noticed that whoever had wallpapered this room had in fact stretched the paper round the corners, creating somewhat of a round corner in a square-cornered room. Well, it had to be done – a little boy very bored with nothing else to do. I pressed firmly into the corner of the wallpaper until it popped, then continued two to three inches, then all the way up as far as I could reach (obviously using the beds did give me an advantage), and I continued to pop the wallpaper up to the height of probably five feet in all four corners (what a good boy I was … not!)

My Nanna was very forgiving generally (especially to me). Unfortunately, my father was not forgiving at all, and I was to be punished for what I had done, most severely. A shame really, because later in life, my Nanna and I used to have a laugh about that particular time and what I had done.

I make no excuses for being a somewhat mischievous child, but looking back, I did have some good reasoning, even if I didn't have the maturity to be able to control many of my actions. Most people would just put it down to 'boys will be boys'.

Another early memory I have would be not obeying my father in his order for me to come down the stairs one time and him telling me if he had to come up those stairs and get me, I'd get 'what for'. My mother tried to remind my father that I was his son and not a recruit in the army, but this had very little effect and I was severely punished again for not obeying my father. He would hit me as hard as he could with a leather slipper – I can still remember how much it used to hurt and sting – and he made me stay in my room without food until he let me come down the next day. As he told my mother, "He will do as he is told, end of." I distinctly remember looking out the window to see if his van would drive away – then I knew I could safely come downstairs.

Basically, most of my memories up to five years old are not very clear, just a constant battle of wills with my father and me obviously losing. I can remember, even at that early age, wanting to escape from this situation, to escape from what should have been a happy home.

One day, I did get free. My father was at work in the local barracks and my mother was preoccupied with my newly-born sister. I took to the street on a red and yellow plastic tractor, but a soldier from my father's barracks stopped and picked me up and returned me (well, never mind – perhaps next time). There were many more attempts to leave the home.

Should a little boy really want to leave the home because he was unhappy at just four years old? Is it possible for such a young child to be unhappy at home if he doesn't know any different?

In these early years, there may have been happier times with my father, but they were so few I do have problems remembering any at all.

***

We moved to Bury St Edmunds and finally moved out of the house where we lived with my Nanna. I actually enjoyed living with my Nanna, even with her three sons still at home. She would always protect me if she could, and because of my Nanna, I felt wanted and loved (at least by her).

(I call her my Nanna as a term simply because she was *my* Nanna – I felt she didn't belong to anyone else. I was very protective of her.) We moved to a council house on a worse estate to where my Nanna's was, and not only a worse estate but the roughest road on that estate as well – that was how desperate my father was to move out of his mother's.

We were living on our own as a family (I use the term loosely) in the house the council had given us, which was a good size, and I did have the luxury of my own bedroom (which was something my father never had with four siblings). But although this was a luxury to those who hadn't had this and came from large families, I personally didn't know any different. But I initially did appreciate have my own space, although this was short-lived when my own space basically turned out to be more of a prison cell than a bedroom. You see, if I played up (or what my father perceived as playing up: not doing what he had ordered me to do), then it was straight to my room as a punishment, most of the time without meals, and not let out until *he* said so. This cell/bedroom was not a place I could have sanctuary in, so I would try to stay out of it as much as possible. In fact, I can remember trying to stay out of the house as much as I could.

At this age I started primary school. I didn't exactly find it easy. You see, with a very strict father (or, as I see it now, a bully for a father), I really did not need to have people bossing me about all day (or that's how I perceived it at the age of five/six), so I struggled with this new environment very much. But on a nicer note, I can remember at that young, tender age being very popular with the girls. Obviously I didn't know much, let alone why I was so popular, but I was and enjoyed this part of school very much (chasing girls that is). Unfortunately, this was a very small part of this new environment and all the other parts seemed to be extremely difficult to deal with.

You would have thought that coming from what you might describe as a regimented home life, I would quite easily fit in with a new regimented environment, but this was not the case. I can remember standing on one of many occasions outside the headmaster's office and thinking *WHY...? Why me? How come I can't just fit in?* (I didn't understand at all). It seemed to me that whatever I did, I would end up in trouble. (It was very confusing, not to mention frustrating). But unfortunately, I hadn't any choice – I *had* to be at school.

I can remember in one of my classes we were doing a project about the sea, and we all had to make something in relation to the sea. I remember going home and telling my parents what we had been asked to do, when my father took over and made a light house. Before you start thinking, *Ah, he was not that bad then, even if a bit strict,* we didn't make this together – he made it. He just took over. And when I took my lighthouse to school, my classmates and my teacher were very impressed. For a while, I was very popular, until it was asked if I had made this on my own. Of course, I said I had because I wanted to fit in.

This scenario happened a number of times as I went through my formative years at school until we were studying the Vikings and again asked to make something memorable. My father really went out there to impress and made me a sword and shield out of wood, rope, and copper. I can remember walking into school that day with my life – sized sword and shield and everyone coming up to me saying, "Wow," and things like "That's cool," but soon, most of the children were telling me I couldn't have made that (and they were right). I was good at art and woodwork, but it was really evident that an adult had had a hand in this, and this situation eventually turned full circle, with my peers saying I was a cheat because my father had done all of the work.

Now as I look back, did he somehow think he owed me? Was he doing it for me or for him? I have drawn my conclusions which will become clear later.

My primary school was not the best of schools, especially for discipline, but the memories I have of my time there aren't really that bad. I can remember learning about the birds and bees, and that was before I was nine years old. But it wasn't from the education department – it was from my peers. At the age of just seven, I can remember some children talking about sex – yes, sex, at seven. Now, in my day, without any internet or mobile phones, etc. (now I sound like an old git or my grandfather – you never think that will happen, but at some point it seems to), seven was an extremely young age to know about sex. My parents hadn't got a clue what I already knew at seven years old. Not a clue.

You see, what was happening was that quite a few parents didn't care what the children saw at all – on TV, videos, magazines, or even as part of real life. Whether this was out of ignorance (and I think there was a lot of it on that estate) or because they just didn't have any sense of decency or morals, we can't be sure. I think there were equal measures of both. (I must add here, a huge part of this story is so relevant to the skill, or rather lack of skill/care, with parenting).

The estate seemed to be full of the kind of people who think it's perfectly acceptable for two mothers to be having a full-on fight out on the front lawn of their house. (When I say 'lawn', I really mean a scabby bit of old dried earth that they called their front garden.) Where it was totally acceptable for the father to spend most of his time in the pub, drinking and fighting. Where old settees and car parts were quite happily strewn across various front gardens (I remember this very well – in the summer of '76 with soaring temperatures, the neighbours dragged their settees and chairs out on the front garden to watch the racing on the TV through the window). Where kids would run across ALL gardens, regardless of who's it was, through hedges, over walls, trampling all the flowers underfoot – a street with people who had no respect for anything or anybody… Wow, what a place to live.

However, there were also a lot of hard-working people with values and some principles, but unfortunately, councils do have a tendency to club together all the rough end of society in one place. I can see why they do this, but with human nature being what it is, there are more people who will drop to the lowest level. Others who are more determined to rise above it will just leave the estate, only for the council to move more of the same in. Then you start to have serious problems, as we did. We had drug deals taking place round the shopping precinct at all times of the day in front of young children. It was a bit like what you might imagine the Bronx area in New York to be like, and bullying was rife. Really, the whole estate was a bigger version of what the schools were like.

I suppose, when I do think back, there were only minor incidents at that school which I guess were starting to shape me for the next school. I mean, even at the ages of five through to nine, I was already very physically confident and could happily hold my own, as I often had to. At that age, it was mainly just name calling, but I can remember building quite a bit of respect (physically) by the time I left that school for the next chapter of my education.

CHAPTER 3

Middle School

It was time to start middle school on the estate in Bury St. Edmunds. This was a rough school to say the least. It seemed as if it had accelerated from the primary school to a totally different level. Most of the teachers in the school were afraid of the pupils, especially the third- and fourth-year students. I remember on my first day the teacher telling the whole class: "Those of you who want to learn, sit on the left of the classroom; those of you who are not bothered, sit on the right." As a ten-year-old boy with quite a few of his peers deciding that the right was the place to be, how could I go to the left? The ridiculing I would have to endure would be immense, but in my heart I knew it was wrong to go with them – I mean, I was at school to learn. Even at that age, I didn't want to end up like one of the thugs and dead-beats that use to walk around that estate, but I also was a painfully shy boy, desperately wanting to fit in and be one of the cool kids, not the weirdo or the boy always on his own, which I did quite often find myself. So which side…? Well, unfortunately, my will to fit in overcame my sensibility, and I sat with the wasters – a group of all boys (what a surprise) who didn't want to learn anything and thought they were cool.

So that's an idea of the type of school I was in. It soon become evident that really, in this place, the students were the ones in charge, not the other way round. There literally were hardly any rules that were abided by and hardly any teachers able to enforce the rules that were in place.

On one occasion in my class, a group of lads was messing about and disrupting the rest of the class quite badly when my male (and that is relevant) teacher lost it. He walked across the classroom and singled out the ringleader (shall we call him Patrick), shouted at the boy, then lifted him onto the table so he was at eye height to the teacher and continued to shout him. Things like: "Do you want to grow up stupid and not ever get a decent job or have anything? Because the way you are going, that is what is going to happen."

Patrick just stood there smirking back at the teacher, and when the teacher had finished his rant, Patrick jumped off the table, and as he ran out of the class, he shouted at the teacher, "You'll pay for that, you bastard."

And pay for it he did. The next day, that teacher wasn't at work and there were rumours going round the school. The following day, we were told he wouldn't be able to take our class, but just then, who should walk in? Yes, the teacher in question, sporting a nice pair of large very dark sun glasses and clearly in some discomfort. During the lesson, the teacher took the sun glasses of to reveal nearly all the left-hand side of his face all battered and bruised. So what the rest of him was like is anybody's guess. Patrick had clearly told one of his uncles what had happened in school and obviously lied that the teacher had picked on him for no reason at all, so his uncle had gone to the school that night and 'taught the teacher a lesson'.

In that school, you basically (as a boy) had two choices – you could either fight or become a very good runner, both of these I managed to excel in. My father always told me: "Stand up for yourself, don't be a coward, stand and fight." (Ironic, really, but more of that later.) He was teaching me what he had learnt in the forces with unarmed combat. So if I was confronted by a bully (or two or three even, because bullies normally like to be in with others and not on their own), I would not run but would fight.

I started to get somewhat of a name for myself. But then the 'one or two lads' were turning into whole gangs of lads, and unless I had started to fight like Bruce Lee, I was in trouble. So the other physical skill came in to play – RUN! And run I did, but definitely not always. I would weigh up the situation and think, *What are my chances here? If I stay and fight, will I be more popular with the other kids?* Then I'd make my decision. (Now, I know the fight or flight emotions in my brain were trying to ascertain the best option, but then my conscious mind would finally win – I had the chance to be someone, even if it was amongst a bunch of delinquents.)

I can also remember being very principled and assuming I had got this behaviour or attitude from my father, to do what was 'right' whatever the consequences. (I would question this thinking later.) Once, I was walking home from school with my best friend (well, I actually mean my *only* friend), who, shall we say, was a bit wimpy and very spoilt as the only son of a couple as old as my Nanna. Suddenly, we were surrounded by youths, probably ten to fifteen of them, all poking and taunting at me and my friend (I will call him Paul.) Me being me, I went to take action. It turned out that they were in fact aiming this abuse at Paul and told me to keep out. One boy then stepped forward and confronted Paul, toe to toe. I can remember my friend's face as he looked back at me, with an expression just asking for help. I stood there and said, "I can't help … not if it's one to one. That wouldn't be fair or right, Paul."

I remember the other boys looking at me as if to say, *What is he going on about?* And with that, the boy toe-to-toe with my best friend hit him, not once but a number of times, until he had blood coming out of his nose and running down his shirt. That was when I stepped in, but not to fight, just to stop it. I just said, "That's enough. He isn't going to fight you, so next time pick on someone who will at least fight back or don't fight at all." For a brief minute, I thought they were all going to start, then I would have had my hands full. I'm not sure what the outcome would have been – I'd probably have run.

On another occasion, yet again I was walking home with another lad from the fourth year, just chatting, when we again were surrounded by a crowd of people. Not one lad came forward but three and started on what seemed to be my new friend (or was he, really?). My principles were that one-to-one was fair, but two- or three-to-one wasn't fair. So I stepped in.

After what seemed to be twenty minutes of fighting (it was probably only two to three minutes), I found myself still standing, helping my new friend up. The teachers came out of the school to intervene at this point. Later, my new friend did admit to me with an apology that he had been bullied by this group for a while and had befriended me because he knew I could take care of myself. I didn't really mind, to be honest, because I didn't have a lot of time for the pupils of that school anyway. This fight was a good excuse to put some bullies in their place, and as it wasn't in the school grounds, I couldn't be punished for it, so to me that was an even better result at the time.

The strange thing now, remembering and looking back, knowing what I know now, is that both the boys who had befriended me were gay (don't get me wrong, I am *not* homophobic by any stretch of the imagination), and I suppose I could see it, I just didn't know what it was about at the time. It may sound odd that when these boys befriended me we must have seemed very different, but I was very shy and I really only had one friend at any time mostly, as I wasn't very popular and would rather just hide away on my own. Well, that's not strictly true – it wasn't what I'd rather do, but it was what came easiest to me due t my personality – that or fight, it seemed.

For a boy with my personality, you would have thought my physical strength would have made me very confident, but it definitely did not. You see, it was one thing fighting in school, but across the estate, well, that was a different situation altogether because you could find yourself with a knife in you; it was that rough. So you would pick carefully where you were going and what you were doing. It did seem to get better as I got older and had more respect. To be honest, it's amazing how I managed to spend six years on that estate without getting stabbed, but I was becoming a lot more confident physically. In fact, due to my schooling, I was very confident in the physical manner, never shying away from a situation that I could have some control in, but mentally,… well, that was a different story entirely. You see, I thought I could control any given situation with a physical response, but as the book progresses, you will see how this mindset was to only make things worse, not better.

Bullying was an everyday event in the school and on the estate. Most of the bullying in the early years, especially at school, was, as I remember, only a physical thing – you would just get poked and pushed about the playground or the playing field until you reacted physically by fighting. I don't remember experiencing any verbal abuse at either of these schools.

At the time, I thought the reason the school bullying was only physical was because of the lack of brain … (Now I know it's more complicated than that.) You see, as I said earlier, all the bullying was from the boys at those schools and hardly any of the boys wanted or were able to learn an education due to the physical bullying they would receive if they (god forbid) went against the anti-learning culture of the school amongst the boys. (There were a few girls who didn't want to learn anything as well, but it was mainly among the boys.) When being pushed from one lad to another with the odd kick thrown in, you very quickly needed to make a decision. One: *Do I fight? If I do, what are my chances of getting out of this situation in one piece and not ending up in hospital?* Or two: *RUN!*

Now for most lads on the receiving end, this was a very easy decision to make. Just run and don't stop for anything till you get home, not even for a teacher. (The chances are, teachers wouldn't be able or willing to get in the middle of a fight between one boy and about ten others.) So just run straight out through the school gates and home.

Me being me (unlike most, I think), I would have to weigh up the situation very quickly. As I've said, I was very physically confident. I would be battling with these thoughts very quickly flashing round my brain – it was as if I could hear a voice (my father's?) saying, "Don't be a coward, stand up for yourself – fight, boy." And the other part, probably the pragmatic part, was saying, "Just run, you really are up against it here." If that was not bad enough, then a third voice would be saying, "What right do they have to bully me? I haven't done anything wrong to them. So *if* I fight and win, then I would have their respect, but do I really want that respect?"

All these questions in a ten-year-old head … To be honest, sometimes I would just run and run until I got home and obviously not tell my father of my actions, and other times I would fight, and without sounding big-headed, I'd normally win in the end. I think even at that age I thought that if I ploughed into these boys, they would think, *What the hell? He must be mad to take ALL of us on.* And then they would start to back off once three or four of them were on the floor. But it would then go the other way, and they would say, "Join us – be part of our gang." So I gained some physical respect but then they would turn again when I would say, "Thanks, but no thanks … I just want to be left alone." (Yet again, what a statement! That was the last thing I wanted, but having said that, even at ten years old, I didn't want to be part of a gang, any gang. So I would keep getting more harassment to join and was constantly asked what was wrong with me. I suppose in a way that was the start of the verbal bullying (name-calling), but at the time it just seemed like harassment.

If I had known that you could make a lot of money by fighting another person, perhaps things would have turned out differently.

With reference to the middle school – in the coming years with a new headmaster, the school did start to get a lot better for its pupils. I just wanted to add that.

CHAPTER 4

The holiday and early visits

For a couple of years in the seventies, we (the whole country) went through hard times, according to my father. But by 1979, when I was nine, my father was now working with his old school friend and earning a good living as a carpenter/builder. So that year, we were told we would be going on holiday *abroad*. The first time on a plane for me, my sister, and mother, and, for reasons that only become apparent a lot later on, my Nanna would be joining us. My father told us we were going to stay in a five-star hotel in Menorca (a small Spanish island in the Mediterranean). Wow, I was going to be going on an aeroplane! This was something that definitely excited me.

Also that year, my father took me on my own (a rare event) to a Honda garage to look at a car he might be interested in (or so I thought at the time). I didn't quite understand why he wanted me there, but there I was in this showroom, looking at all these brand new shiny cars and smelling that smell that you only get from a showroom – I never forgot that smell and can remember as the salesman gave my dad the keys to a new Honda Prelude. How excited and proud I felt! (No matter how much of a strict and unloving drunk he was at the time, I could still be proud and think of him as my father.) I thought, *My father is buying a brand new car, and not just any car*. Honda, at the time, were not really known in the UK for cars, more for motorcycles.

I couldn't believe it. And then a few weeks later, this metallic red Honda Prelude pulled up in front of our house with my father at the wheel. I remember running out to get a closer look and hopefully a ride, especially in the front.

At this time, I hadn't realised that my father was even interested in cars. As a little boy, I was mad on the things, absolutely loved them – from Matchbox, Corgi, or Dinky … I had books on cars, magazines; in fact everything I could get would be in association with cars. I used to just sit in my parents' car and look out of the window or watch how it was being driven. And now I thought my father was interested in cars after all, buying the Honda. At last we had something in common. Up to that point, I just felt I annoyed him all the time. But he wasn't really interested in cars at all.

So in 1979, we were on holiday in Menorca after picking up this brand new car. Wow, what a year, thinking how well my father was doing and being so proud (but me never being one to gloat – just like my mother). But perhaps these things weren't having the effect that my father had wished for.

Being in Menorca with my Nanna was great as she kept me very close, and I enjoyed that closeness, as I didn't get that from either of my parents. It was my Nanna who showed me love and affection and also made me and others laugh. Really that came through her lack of thinking. My Nanna was far from stupid – in fact, under different circumstances, she could probably have done very well for herself with a good education. But I guess they were different times during and after the war. (I nearly said, "During the war ..." like old Uncle Albert of *Only Fools and Horses*. Bless him, I would love to have an Uncle Albert ...) Anyway, my Nanna just wouldn't think first before jumping in.

On one occasion, that is literally what she did. We had arrived back at the harbour from a boat trip and the Spanish escort shouted to everyone on the open boat, "Please leave the boat this end." Suddenly, my Nanna decided, for reasons only known to her, to literally jump off the other end of the boat that by now had drifted about six feet from the dockside. An unknown gentleman grabbed hold of my Nanna's arms just as she was about to drop into the water. That little incident had the whole boat in laughter, except the Spanish escort, who just looked somewhat bemused.

Another time she (and God only knows how, let alone why) got her bra trapped in the hotel lift and we had to call maintenance to free it as it was stalling the lift from functioning properly. What a woman! And I loved her for it.

I found out a few years later that the reason my father had asked his mother on holiday with us was in fact so he could keep sloping off to get drunk. He did that on a number of occasions on that holiday, as usual causing trouble, sometimes in the hotel, so when we walked into the dining hall, we would get looks as if to say, "Oh, you're the family with the troublemaking drunk father." What could have been lovely holiday was spoilt by my father and his behaviour, which he never made any apologies for.

My father had a serious drink problem, but was very cunning at covering it from people. Back at home on the estate, he would leave work about 5.30 pm, dropping off his work partner at home (let's call him Mr Dingle). Then he would go with a load of new mates to a pub, then on to a club, because in those days clubs could stay open later, especially private ones. (Where they really mates? The only thing they all had in common was the fact that they loved to drink, and when I say drink, I mean drink until unconsciousness set in or money ran out – now, where have we heard that before?)

My father – and I remember this like it was yesterday – would get himself so drunk that he could hardly walk but somehow used to unfortunately find his way home. He would literally crawl up the stairs, then stagger and fall his way down the landing until he got to my bedroom. By now, my heart would be pounding so hard it felt as if it would burst out of my chest at any given moment. I would just lie there praying, and when I say praying, I mean hands clenched, looking up to the ceiling, saying, "Please God don't let him in here, not again, pleeease." I couldn't have begged more for this to stop.

Now, if you're thinking he touched me inappropriately, then you would be wrong. It wasn't anything like that. Pulling me about was a favourite, especially round the head, telling me I needed to be a man (what, like him? I don't think so) and also telling me stories of his time in the forces. Now, I will prepare you for this because it is sick, and there were many stories like this that he told me at the age of nine and ten, in my bed at two, three, or four in the morning. He once told me that he and some other soldiers in a place called Aden in the Middle East went down to the local village at night time and set a number of detonators in this huge pile of rubbish that the locals used to wade through, looking for food or anything they could use or sell. Then the soldiers all retreated to a safe distance where they could watch as the rubbish heap blew up. He told me how he and his mates would be laughing, seeing these dead bodies lying everywhere, limbs missing. Even at the age of nine and ten I found this sickening. If he thought I would think he was cool or a hard man for carrying out these atrocities, he was seriously mistaken. Even then, I really couldn't believe that my father would be telling me and laughing about it like it was something to be proud of.

That was when I began to stop looking up to my father. Your father is someone you should be proud of – every little boy wants to think his father is superman, not an evil monster. And the worst of it all is that, because he was inebriated at the time, he could never remember the poison that he was telling me. And it got worse, but I'm not prepared to go into any further depraved descriptions. It's not right, and even if that is the sort of thing the armed forces get up to, it definitely isn't the sort of bedtime stories that a ten-year-old needed or should hear.

This was happening two to three times a week. I hated the stories, I hated the smell of alcohol on his breath as he made me listen, I hated him, but I was also just a boy who was scared witless of him; I mean, really scared to the point of peeing myself under the bed sheets. He was full of venom and hatred, telling me that all people were scum and they needed putting in their place – so much hatred, anger, and bitterness, and all of this poison he was feeding his ten-year-old son. After eighteen months of this, suddenly on a mid-week evening, drunk as usual, he was pulled over by the police and breathalysed. He was subsequently taken to court, where he lost his licence for eighteen months. Obviously this didn't stop him drinking. However, he did stop coming in drunk to my room at two or three in the morning. I couldn't have been happier that this abuse could finally end.

But now he had to rely on other people in the family to drive him around – his two younger brothers (he worked with them during this time) and also my mother. At weekends, to get off the estate that he hated so much (that was the only reason he took us as a family anywhere), my mother would have to drive, which in itself caused a huge number of arguments because' my father was (and is, at the time of writing) a very arrogant man and extremely opinionated. So if my mother did *anything* out of place, or what he considered to be wrong, they would start arguing – or rather, he would start bullying.

Although my mother was quite submissive in some ways, in others, she could argue for Britain, and when my father was sober, she would argue the toss with him over any given subject. (It used to drive me mad, this constant arguing, bickering, and then silences, especially after a drinking session.) I really don't have any memories of a family occasion where we would all be together with laughter – the only time I can recall any family outings with any form of laughter was if my Nanna was present.

What I can remember about going out in the car is feeling very isolated and alone sitting in the back seat. My sister would constantly put herself in the middle of the two front seats, which really annoyed me as it meant I couldn't see the driver, whether it be my mother or father. I just wanted to be able to see the craft of driving a car, but my sister would always be in the way and getting the complete attention of both my parents.

I must add, this was the norm anyway. You are probably thinking that I was just jealous, and you'd be right … Yes, I was jealous, because although there were four in this family unit, to me it felt more like there were three and one (me). You see, my sister was the apple of my father's eye (his little girl, as he would say). My mother, because of the closeness she had with her own mother, had a close bond with my sister. Where was there any room for a little boy in this equation?

To be honest, most of the time in my formative years, at home or in the back seat of the car with my sister, was spent arguing anyway. It was like a whole house full of arguments, parents, and siblings. Argue! Argue! Argue! All the time. Which is why I used to try to spend as much of my time away as possible from the so-called home environment. My sister knew she had the whip hand with my parents and used that position as much as she could. I remember on many occasions when my sister and I would be in the lounge with the television on and suddenly, for no reason at all (or no reason I could see then), she would scream and shout my name and tell me to get off her, even though I wasn't near her. Some would say, "Well, that's brothers and sisters for you." But she was always pulling this stunt, which was alright when it was just my mother in the house because all my mother would do is come through and shout at me, "Leave your sister alone," but never follow it up with any sort of punishment. She found it very amusing when I was told off – she would sit there grinning, but not letting either one of my parents see her reaction – very devious girl my sister was. But if my father was at home and she did it, that was a different matter. His slipper would come off, and it was then a race as to how quickly I could get out of his way before that leather slipper careered round my back end or even worse, round the tops of my thighs.

He was quite proud of telling people about when I was a little boy and didn't do as I was ordered (and I say 'ordered' because that's what it was – it was not requested, it was an order! "Do this or else", and a lot of the time I got the 'or else'). When I was only one or two years old and had a nappy under my trousers, that would cushion the blow of the slipper, so wouldn't give the intended impact. My father got round this situation by simply hitting me with the slipper at the top of my thighs, under the nappy or pant line, for a greater impact. And boy, it worked. It use to sting like hell, especially if I had not been a quick as I wanted and had copped a number of these whacks.

Another thing my father seemed to be proud of was when I was two years old. People say these are the 'terrible twos', and I know there must be some truth to that, but I think the way my father behaved towards me was actually making me resilient to the punishments and more determined to prove him wrong, even at that early age. My father would put me into my cot and wanted me to sleep. I, obviously not wanting to go to sleep, would climb over the cot and get out of the room. So my father, after this happening a number of times, decided enough was enough and decided to actually tie me to the cot. I would then be completely restrained and totally unable to move. As an extra measure, he would screw the door handle on upside down so I couldn't get out of the room, even if I'd worked out how to get myself untied.

CHAPTER 5

A new school

At the age of eleven my parents had sold the ex-council house and we were moving to a village about four miles from Bury St Edmunds called Culford. Finally, my father had got what he wanted, and we were now off the estate and in a village. For my sister and me, this meant starting a new school halfway through the middle schooling years in a Church of England school.

So there we were in a new village, and I didn't know anyone at all. I remember as if it were yesterday walking down the village to the school bus stop where there were about ten other children of various ages from nine to sixteen. As I got onto the bus, I looked at one of the lads, who was, shall we say, quite a large boy, and he said, "Hello." At the time this was reassuring, considering nobody else had spoken, but being a shy boy, I elected to sit on my own, on the same side of the bus just behind the big lad. After just sitting down, suddenly another lad stood right in front of me and told me I was in his seat. Now, this was strange as the bus was hardly full and there were plenty of other seats. But the lad obviously wanted the seat that I had elected to sit on and was very willing to physically show how much he wanted it.

As I've said before, physical confidence was not a problem at all for me, so after a bit of pushing and shoving, I took a firm hold of him and put him on the floor of the bus. With my foot firmly at the lad's throat, I said, "What is your problem with me sitting here?" As I said this, I removed my foot and let him get to his feet. He grunted, shuffled to the back of the bus, and sat there in the middle of the back seat like a king on his throne with his subjects to either side. I thought, *Great, that's a good start to the new school – I haven't even got into the place and I've already had a fight.*

Now as it turned out the large lad I had said "Hello" to (Kris) started to tell me who I had just put on the floor of the bus. Apparently, it was the "toughest boy in the school", but I just sarcastically said, "Oh good!" I really did not need this. I was scared enough starting a new school, let alone making enemies on the first day.

You would think after bruising the ego of a bully, he would just keep out of my way. But oh no – instead, this boy wanted me to join him and his gang. I told him defiantly, "No, all I want is to be left alone," but still he kept befriending me. So I thought, *Well, I'd rather just let him think I'm his friend and then he will stop bothering me to join his gang.* So we actually did spend some time together and had a sort of mutual understanding: *You leave me alone and I'll leave you alone.*

But underneath, as I found out, he was not happy about the new boy embarrassing him in front of others and was holding a huge angry grudge against me. I found this out one day on the playing field when he came at me from behind and got a very strong hold round my neck. I actually thought he was going to strangle me as he kept tightening his hold – I was literally gasping for breath and getting weaker. I knew I'd really have to go mad to get him off me. Looking back, I don't think for one minute he knew just how close he was to completely stopping me from being able to breathe. Just as I was about to pass out through lack of oxygen, I lifted him up and over my head and we both crashed onto the grass. Now I was the one with him in my hands, holding on. This sent him mad as a dog, and it took everything I had to get control of him. Needless to say, eventually, I was able to walk away and we did not speak for a number of weeks after that altercation.

I was trying to get used to this new school, but I'm afraid, coming from a school with no rules, this Church of England school was like a prison to me. They had lines up the middle of the corridors, like we were the cars on a main road. There were so many rules I would always end up in trouble one way or the other, mostly because I was not used to this system – or that was what I thought at the time.

At this school I was put in a class with a lovely teacher (or so I thought at the time). She happened to be an old school friend of my Nanna's. I thought, *This is a result*. When visiting my Nanna a few days after starting the school, she said she'd had a chat with my new teacher (who we will call Mrs Temple), and Mrs Temple said she would look after me as I was special. This was initially very comforting for a shy boy such as me and especially as I was starting the school as a complete newbie in the third year.

In the first week or so, I just tried to keep my head down and see if I could make a friend or two, which I found really difficult to do being so shy. I'd already met the big lad from the bus, who, I found out, they all called Beefy, and the other lad who hated my guts for embarrassing him not once but twice. This was not looking good for me at all. When we had a break time, I would just find somewhere quiet and sit on my own with my own thoughts, praying in my head that I would wake up and all of this would be a bad dream.

I did however befriend a lad, but as with Beefy, he wasn't in my form class either. In fact, I wasn't really friends with anyone in my form class at all – I just didn't fit in. The only time anyone really wanted to be mates was when I was fighting another boy (they felt safe with me). Fighting did occur a little too often due to a reputation following me from my previous school. I was at the time one of the tallest in the year, if not in the school, and although I was very slim, I was also muscular. So the old adage that people pick on the smallest isn't always true! In fact, I was being picked on or challenged nearly daily in the first few months of being at the new school and this was creating a persona that I really didn't want and definitely didn't need.

I remember one occasion well. Because I could easily defend myself against one or even two boys at the same time (don't get me wrong – I'm not being big-headed, and fighting isn't something to be proud of unless you are in a ring, getting paid vast amounts of money for it), I was grabbed behind the woodwork block one day by a whole gang of about ten lads, all shouting, "Just how tough are you?" All ten or so of them were kicking and punching at the same time. Then they held me up against the wall of the building with a sash window directly behind my head. One of the gang decided to run down the playground and leap at my face with his fist clenched like Superman.

When I saw what was about to happen, with all my strength I pulled my right arm away from the boys holding it against the wall. To protect myself from the Superman boy, I put it up in front of my face but outstretched with the palm facing outward, with the arm fully extended.

Well, this boy hit my hand and dropped like a stone to the floor, where he just lay without any movement at all. All the other lads suddenly all disappeared and in the same moment I thought I'd killed him. He just lay there for what seemed like hours, but it was probably no more than one minute. Luck was never on my side, so when this happened, I thought, *That's it, now I'll end up in Borstal or something.* I remember two teachers coming across the playground and the first one shouting at me to get to the Head's office. The other teacher was holding the boy when suddenly there he was, still alive! I felt such a relief as he sat with the teacher just blankly gazing around, somewhat bemused at what had just happened.

All of a sudden there was another bellow from the male teacher: "I thought I told you to get to the Headmaster's office!"

I'd already spent quite a lot of time in the headmaster's office. But this time, I was just relieved that the boy was still alive.

I was physically bullied for the best part of that year, but in the end, I think they were running out of boys to fight with me. In a later year, though, there was another incident. We had a sports day. I was in the boys' toilet minding my own business when all of a sudden the boy I'd had an altercation with on the bus on day one burst in with two lads, one under each arm, and asked me to take one of them and flush his head in the toilet . I said, "No, leave me out of this," and received a mouthful of expletives from the bully boy as I left him to it and ran out of the toilets. I kept thinking even at that age, say twelve or so, *What is it with these people I'm surrounded with? Why can't they just leave me be?*

Physical bullying was something I could deal with, the only trouble being that if you were always the last boy standing, you were also the one who would take all the blame and all the punishment too. I always thought, then and now, that this was very unfair, but I think the teachers were just looking for the easiest scapegoat and didn't, in my experience, want to hear reasons for what they just saw as boys fighting. This was very unfortunate for me and something that I seemed to just have to deal with. So I did – by trying to avoid conflicting situations as much as possible.

On the other hand, you have mental bullying, and this one I

really struggled with. In fact, to be honest, I didn't deal with the mental bullying well at all. It wasn't just the constant name calling either; it was the psychological aspect of the bullying that I couldn't understand as a boy of twelve Oh boy, children can be very vicious.

You see, one thing I can see and understand now as an adult is that bodily abuse heals. If someone hits you in the face and you end up with a black eye, within a week or two, it will have healed up and anyone looking at you wouldn't know you even had a black eye. But the memory scar will remain with you till the day you die, and that's the hard one to deal with. It's always the memory that haunts us all, and even if you possess the temperament for forgiveness, it cannot be erased from your memory, ever! As a coping strategy, most people, as my mother did, push these events to the back of their mind/memory and try not to think about it again (easier said than done for some people).

Halfway through that first year, physical bullying was replaced with verbal bullying. It started with name calling. To this day, I could never understand how or why my peers decided to call me the name they had chosen. You see, my name at school was different to what it is now – then, my surname was Davies, and the kids used to call me Duggy, which I was very upset with. "Duggy! Duggy! Duggy Davies!" is all I would hear, mainly from a small selection of boys, but some others would also join in from time to time. I just couldn't seem to get away from the constant barrage of this name-calling, and because the only way I knew to deal with this sort of bullying was to either fight or run, that's exactly what I would do. I started missing school (in those days they called it bunking off), so if I knew I had a class with those boys, I just wouldn't attend. I would go and find somewhere to hide around the school grounds.

This behaviour started to have an impact on my schooling, and it was only going to get worse. One day, I'd had just about enough of these morons. I had double art coming up that afternoon, and not only was I good at it, I also enjoyed it, so I actually *wanted* to be in class. So I found all three of the lads, one at a time though, and using one of my strengths (pardon the pun), had this boy in a ... shall we say, firm grip. Firstly, I asked him what his problem was with me and why on earth he kept calling me Duggy. Where did the name come from? I asked him a number of questions which were obviously a bit too complicated for all three of them because none of them could answer. Incidentally, many years later, I was speaking with one of the name-calling culprits and asked him then, after nearly twenty years, to tell me why, and he couldn't answer then either. So I just said sarcastically, "Well, that explains everything doesn't it?" To which he replied, "Sorry I don't understand." And I said, "No, exactly."

Basically, they were just so immature they didn't even know themselves why they were literally torturing another lad with this constant bullying, and they didn't even realise what effect it was having at all – pure ignorance. I feel sure many of you out there had similar experiences.

I really wish I could say that was the end of it (the end of the verbal bulling), but unfortunately it wasn't. Not only did these three continue until we moved to the next school, but some girls also thought it might be fun to humiliate me. They told me that one of the most desired girls in the school had 'the hots' for me (I will call her Claire) and would like to get to know me better. So I wrote a letter to her. I thought I'd hit the jackpot. 'But I was still a shy young man and not confident around anyone, especially girls – in fact, they frightened the life out of me. So here we are – letter written.

The girls who told me of Claire's interest kept very close to me throughout this whole charade. And that's exactly what it was. The day came when I finally found enough courage to speak to Claire. Just as I was about to speak, the lead girl in this charade shouted out that it had just been a wind up and Claire didn't even know who I was. Added to this, they then passed the letter I had written around the whole year group.

Well, I was mortified to say the least, and the embarrassment stayed with me for a very long time, not to mention the question 'Why?' Why did these girls do this? What had I done to them to deserve this deception and cruelty? I never did get any answers and my confidence plummeted to even deeper levels, if that was at all possible.

CHAPTER 6

Growing up ... a bit too fast

When I was eleven years old, I had started to shave daily. This was something I found incredibly difficult to deal with because how on earth could I cover it up? At this time, I didn't think my adult life was just starting. I thought my whole life was just finishing. And then it got even worse because I started growing hair in other places as well as my face. How much worse could it get – a painfully shy lad growing hair, looking more like a man instead of a boy? How on earth was I going to deal with this?

Well, in truth, I wasn't and I didn't. In fact, I think at that time in my life, I had developed the first symptoms of depression. I really couldn't see a way out of this and felt totally out of control.

So there I was at school, after running the old electric razor round my face in the morning (incidentally, it was my father's electric razor and I didn't dare tell him I was using it), hoping and praying nobody would notice the fact that I was shaving, because if they did ... all hell would break loose. My fellow peers could give me enough abuse without this. As it happens, I didn't get any abuse about shaving, but the other areas that had decided to sprout hair did become a problem; a serious problem.

As I said before, thanks to my previous school, I excelled in two areas – fighting, which the school was definitely not interested in, and running, which the school *was* interested in.

Now! Being very good at running was ok, but I was good at most sports that didn't involve a team (I know – there is no I in team). It wasn't intentional, it was just that the other players, for whatever reason, didn't want me to be part of their team. Perhaps they felt threatened by me, I don't know!

I wasn't really into team sports anyway as I had trouble relying on others, who I felt would let me down (there's a little insight into my somewhat complicated character – more about that very soon). But it was still very upsetting being forced by the teachers to play, with everyone passing to one another but never passing to me.

I remember once when I was on the sports field and was meant to be playing rugby with the other lads, but as usual was being left out, so I just stood (freezing cold, I might add) on my own on the pitch, away from all the action, bored to the bone. As I was standing there, the rugby teacher (a stocky Welsh man) shouted at me, "Boy, join in, come on, play the game!"

Well, I attempted to join the game, but to no avail – no passing. I might as well have been invisible or a ghost – it was always a waste of time. But the teacher obviously had other ideas, bellowing at me again. "Join in, boy – what's your problem?" That was just the question I needed. I thought it was an ideal time to tell this teacher what my problem was, and so I did. After taking a big deep breath, I proceeded to explain that I did not know why the other lads didn't want me to play with them as a team – no matter how hard I tried, they wouldn't have me join in. What he said was, and I quote: "If the boys don't let you in, then push in. Just push your way in and take control."

So that's exactly what I did. I ran into the group of lads as they were all trying to tackle one other and I grabbed the ball and ran – and boy, did I run – right to the end of the pitch and put the ball down. The second time I took the ball from one of the lads and did the same as before, the reaction was quite a bit different, because, you see, I wasn't bothered about which side I was on. I was just trying to make a point, so the first try was at one end and the second was at the other. The teacher bellowed again in my direction, "Boy, which side are you on?"

I shouted back, "I don't know, sir!" Sides…? I'd never had hold of the ball before so I hadn't really paid a lot of attention to who or what the sides were. I came off the pitch and said to the teacher, "I did what you said, and if I hadn't, I still would be left standing on my own, wouldn't I, sir? But I'll never be part of the team if none of them let me, will I, sir?"

I found out later that the teacher had tried to get the rest of the team to let me in more by explaining that if I was one of the fastest boys in the school, they should use the skills I had. And that worked … sort of. The next thing I knew, I was being passed to and was asked to play for the school.

"Hooray!" I hear you say, "What a nice ending." I wished so as well, but … no. I was playing but still on my own. The teacher had said "Use him", and that's exactly what happened. Now, he might have had the best intentions for me, and I'd like to think he thought that if I was playing then perhaps it would evolve into a team participation, but it never did. (I hasten to add, that teacher had no idea of the other problems I was suffering at the time.) So I scored the tries, and there were many – not because I was good at rugby or the team were good, just because I was very fast and nobody could catch me. I used to have the pitch ahead all on my own, so I ended up on my own playing for the team. Ironic, really.

***

So I'd been playing rugby and the summer season was coming around again, and athletics was on the agenda. Running was my thing, (but only over short distances – I absolutely hated cross country), but not just running – I was also good at long jump, high jump, javelin, discus, shot put ... (I was rubbish at hurdles – I think I was running too fast for my legs to take on any other instructions!) But all in all, very good at most sports that didn't involve a team.

The unfortunate part was that to do sports required a change of clothing. Now the problem appears – not the clothing, but the changing part, because changing was exactly what my body had decided to do with some speed as well. I mean, if it wasn't bad enough having to shave at the very young age of eleven, now there was hair appearing everywhere. By the time I was twelve years old, the only part of my body that wasn't covered with hair was my chest (but that happened later). I was a very, very shy young man and definitely didn't have the robustness that would have been required to deal with the barrage of insults and abuse that I suffered for the two years I was at that middle school.

I remember the sports and PE timetable well, even now. Tuesday from 1.30pm to end of school was sports, and Friday was PE (physical education) from 10.30am to 11.30am. Sports were normally on the playing field, and PE was normally in the assembly hall.

My Tuesday went one of two ways. After lunch, I would go straight to the, say, French class before any other pupils and would be waiting first in line to get a seat as close to the door as I could for a quick exit (all had to be planned). So French is over (hooray!) and I'm out of that classroom like a greyhound straight to the changing rooms, actually running to get there before anyone else (and remember, running in corridors was strictly prohibited in that school, but the risk was worth it). I could then get changed and into my sports kit before any of the other lads could start on me.

So there I would be in my long track suit bottoms, even in the height of summer. This did cause some difficulties for me as well, because when I started wearing them, suddenly we had a change of sports teacher who was more of a stickler for the rules. The teachers obviously didn't talk to each other, well, not about the pupils anyway, because I got asked in front of all the other boys why in the height of summer I was wearing long bottoms. I just stood there looking glum and feeling petrified inside with my heart racing, because how on earth could I answer that question? I really don't remember saying anything; there wasn't anything I could say.

Then the worst happened and the teacher said (I'll never forget it), "It's lovely and sunny out there, so go and get a pair of shorts and I'll see you outside in five."

Oh shit, what the hell was I to do? So many thoughts rushing round my brain. *How am I going to get out of this? If I run, the teacher will know I'm missing, but if I get the shorts, then the other boys will start on me.* What a dilemma. So I chose the latter and hoped for the best, which I fully knew wasn't going to happen, but at least the teacher would then know why I wore long bottoms. Well, that was my theory anyway. It did not work though. The teacher didn't hear or chose not to hear the abuse I was getting – the little one liners behind his back. I thought *That's the last time that's going to happen*, and over the next few weeks I would move to plan b for the sports lesson.

On Tuesday, in the after-lunch French lesson, I wasn't in first this time, and wasn't sitting near the door either – no need. Because as we all came out of the French classroom and everyone turned left, I went right; in fact, right out of the school grounds completely, through the park, and into the local graveyard to eat the lunch I'd saved (basically for something to do). I would just sit there or have a walk around and read the headstones. Later, I'd move closer to the school exit and wait until I saw at least a dozen children come out of the school grounds. Then I would join the rest through the hedge and get on the bus home as normal.

This went on for a number of weeks when suddenly we were told that in future there would be a register called before sports lessons. That was not what I wanted to hear – how on earth was I going to get round this problem? Well, when the next sports lesson was due, I'd had a bad morning of name-calling as it was and I thought, *I couldn't give a toss if there is a register to be called. I'm still not going to sports.* And I didn't. But I also didn't hear anything about not being there either. This was strange – not attending sports lessons even with a register being called, but not being caught for it.

Later, a friend told me how I was getting away with it. My mate Kris and another lad, who I had just thought of as an acquaintance, had been shouting, "Yes" to my name at the sports lesson register. What a mate … a true friend. They both knew I was going through a hard time with the other boys, but neither of them knew what it was like because they were not maturing at the rate I was. (*Blimey*, I thought, *at this rate, if my body doesn't slow down, I'll be an old man before I leave school.*) The trouble was, neither the teachers nor my parents were aware of what was happening. Well, that was about to change.

***

After thirteen (unlucky for some) weeks of not showing for sports lessons, I was walking through the park on my way back to the school to catch the bus when I inadvertently met my form teacher. After an awkward moment, I ran away to catch the bus. I thought at least I'd be able to say why I was truanting, and perhaps the school might give me a concession so I could continue with on with the subject I was very good at.

That didn't happen though. What did happen was that the next morning, my form teacher asked me to stay behind to speak with her. If you remember, she knew my Nanna, so I thought this could turn out ok. How wrong I was. She said she wouldn't say anything to get me in trouble because there was obviously an issue that need addressing. Well, that was reassuring after I'd just told a relative stranger about some very personal details. The next thing I knew, I was being escorted to the Head's office, where I would get the chance to go through the whole story again, not just with him but also with my parents. That's just what I needed – my father involved. As you've probably guessed, nothing changed for me, and I was punished for playing truant.

For a few weeks, I attended sports lessons. One day, a combination of incidents happened that seemed to sum up the confusion in my life. The sports teacher (ironically, the same one who had given me grief over my sports kit) came over to me and expressed an interest in my running. Actually, he said, "Why don't you use your arms when you run?"

This question confused me … Use my arms? I can remember thinking *I run with my legs.* (How ignorant, or is that being unfair? I was only twelve … even though I looked thirty.) *How would I use my arms?* Just as he said those words, I could see all the other boys careering down the sports field toward the changing rooms. Then I panicked – all I could think about was getting into those changing rooms before all the other boys, so I wouldn't have to endure more of the bullying. But the teacher seemed very excited about me.

I said, "Sir, I said I have to go," but he wasn't listening, so I just ran off the field (remember, I was the fastest in the school) and got to the front of the group of boys.

I was just running along the corridor and about to turn in to the changing rooms when I heard the words, "Laddy, come here, NOW!" My heart was racing so fast I could barely draw breath. I knew I was now in trouble (again). The voice belonged to Mrs Reed, the deputy Head – a very strict and angry old Irish woman who took no prisoners.

As I went to her, I could see out of the corner of my eye all the boys going into the changing rooms. What a cow! She had no idea what anguish and pain she had now caused me. I would rather have written a five-hundred-word essay on any subject every day than have to keep going through the same mental torture every week, because they were relentless with it – week in, week out, those horrible little boys would keep pointing and jibing and verbally abusing me (and that's exactly what they were – immature, irresponsible, rude, weak little boys).

As an adult, I know that, but at the time I wasn't mature enough to be able to see it and definitely not mature enough to shrug it off or even verbally attack them back, not mentally. So after being chastised by Mrs Reed, I was told to go. But where? I wasn't going into the changing rooms, not now they were full of boys, so I went into the toilet just down the corridor until just before the final bell. I then ran back into the changing rooms, which were nearly empty, and quickly changed into my uniform just in time to catch my bus home. But it was close.

This sports teacher obviously kept an eye on me, because the next lesson, he came over to speak to me again. What he said totally shocked me. He reckoned he could see a serious runner in me and he offered to teach me how to use my whole body for running. He asked what my best time was currently, and when I told him, he seemed to get even more excited than before. He said, "Just imagine your time if you used the rest of your body, as at the moment you're just running with your legs." He told me to speak to my parents and said he would happily chat to them if they had any doubts about his intentions.

But I never spoke to my parents about this, for two reasons. First, because of a conversation I'd had with an uncle about athletes, who said they didn't earn anything. In those days, it was true; they didn't earn a lot of money – they really pursued their chosen sport for the medals and the recognition of representing their country. As a young man, one thing I did like was collecting money! (I know that sounds a strange way of putting it because it's really saving, but I didn't know that terminology at the time and it felt to me more like collecting.) So when I found out that athletics didn't pay well, or sometimes at all, I wasn't interested. What a mistake. I mean, the reason the teacher was so interested was that just running with legs only and arms waving about, I was still capable of a time of 12.5 seconds for the one hundred metre sprint (bear in mind that the world record at the time was only around 10 seconds).

Second, even if I had told my parents, I know my father would have told me I needed to get a proper job And my mother, well, she didn't really show any opinions, at least not when it came to my education. Now I look back and think, *If only*, but it didn't happen. My decision, my regret (no blame).

I was so frustrated with this whole situation … I mean, I was good at something, really good, But I didn't have the capacity to cope with the situation I felt the other boys were putting me in. And the people around me, parents and teachers (who, I might add, are meant to care for children), just weren't interested.

The other problem was the more I played truant and got away with it, the more times I did it. There were classes that I didn't really like, maybe because of the teacher or because I knew a group of lads would verbally pick on me. Or they would keep passing pieces of paper with abuse on them up and down the class until they got to me. I felt completely trapped in these classes because, as I said before, my way of dealing with it was to physically fight back, but sitting in a classroom with a teacher present, I could do nothing except just get more and more upset. This would manifest itself as anger, but I was completely paralysed in that environment and would have to just wait until the lesson had finished, when these boys knew what was coming to them.

Often, they would hold back with the teacher, asking questions about the subject we were meant to be learning, keeping her or him occupied until I had no choice but to leave before them. Then I would be late for the next class and told off again. This situation happened on a regular basis and got me in a huge amount of trouble – nearly every Friday lunchtime I would be in detention, which meant only having ten minutes for lunch. I just felt like I wanted to run away, but where would I go? I was trapped completely. One positive for being in detention every week was on that day, which was a Friday, I could have a large school dinner, simply because, as I was the last to get to the food hall, I could (if I liked what was on offer) have seconds and thirds sometimes. The rest of the week I would have a packed lunch due to the versatility, especially on days of playing truant, and I always had a healthy appetite.

So there you go – the one thing that I could excel in I kept missing because of bullying. Because indoor PE was another bone of contention for the same reasons (the changing room scenario), I would miss that lesson too. Because the same group of boys were in several different lessons, I would often have to miss some other lessons (including maths), and that definitely didn't help with my education. Not being comfortable in the school environment, my schoolwork really suffered, and hence my grades for the basic subjects were not what they could have been. Accompanied by a miserable home life, I really did struggle with my schooldays.

CHAPTER 7

13 years to 16 years old (the bullying goes on, and on, and on …)

Well …! What can I say – did things get better? I wish. Instead, things just changed – at least, at school they did. I had moved to the upper school (our final school). Let's just say, it didn't get off to a great start.

I felt that nobody knew me – that was a blessing as much as a curse. On the first day, whilst talking to a girl in the classroom, I was suddenly grabbed from behind and dragged from my stool. It wasn't long before I left my attacker on the floor (seconds, if I remember rightly). He claimed to be the girl's boyfriend, and I just thought, *Here we go again, a scuffle on my first day.* It was like history repeating itself.

Again, this may seem like a very trivial thing to happen, and it's probably happened to many of you reading this, but this sort of (as I interpreted it) bad luck did nothing for my **minds** health, which was already fragile at this point from family life and schooling. You see, it wasn't just a scuffle. This boy that I had now sorted out was known as the toughest in his previous school, and now I was again up on offer. This was something I *really* did not need, but on the positive side (although, I might add, I had huge trouble seeing any positive side at that time in my life), the name-calling had stopped. Hooray, that was a great relief, as that was probably the hardest for me to deal with, requiring a mental perspective and not a head lock.

This first year was better than previous school years, but then it could not really have got any worse. I had a few physical altercations, which was fine by me as this was my strong area, and pretty soon was being left alone. The changing room problem from my previous school wasn't so much of a problem anymore as there was a significant increase in the number of boys who looked a bit more like me.

The thing I didn't understand (and as a fifty-year-old man, I still do not understand) is if you are not strong enough at a subject like English, then why on earth put someone through two and a half hours a week trying to learn French? Surely it would be better if all of those like myself had sat in on extra English classes? (Mind you, I wouldn't have thought that at the time, I have no doubt!) It also doesn't seem right to have to do a subject that you really don't like and therefore were not really any good at. How about swapping with another child who feels the same as you do about another subject? Or was it a case of liking it because you were good at it? Psychology again.

**

This first year at school might have been a lot better, but unfortunately, home life was not. I was getting on my bicycle most nights and biking from the village we lived in four miles to the nearest town, Bury St. Edmunds. I would sit on the cross bar perched up against a bollard and watch the cars go round the roundabout in front of me. I can remember thinking on many occasions, *I wonder where they are going; just home or off on a journey?* I really couldn't wait to get behind the wheel of a car and to finally have what I saw as freedom and my own space.

It's alright being told by your parents that you are really lucky having your own bedroom instead of sharing with other siblings, and I do understand that, but when that room is in a house of discomfort and misery, it really doesn't matter that it's your own room – in fact, it was a very lonely place to be. If I was in that room, all I would hear would be my parents arguing or silence when my mother wasn't talking to my father. On top of that, I was very vulnerable in that room, with only one door and a roof window – if my father came in drunk, I had nowhere to go to escape him. So I tried to stay out of the so-called family home as much as I could. Whilst I was out and on my bike, it was a sort of freedom.

Another thing my father would say, and in this case my mother would back him (it wasn't common for my mother to back him up; not when he was sober), would be how lucky I was because he would take us on holidays, as opposed to my parents, who had never had holidays. But for the first two to three days of each holiday, my father would be miserable and grumpy, not wanting to do anything with the family at all. Even at the age of thirteen, I did get the feeling that we were an inconvenience to him and he would rather be on his own. Sure enough, the following day, he would disappear and go on a bender (a term used for someone who goes off hard drinking), and God only knows what would happen then.

It was in 1983 when this happened again. He had booked a holiday in Majorca in an apartment that his own cousin owned, and he was, as usual, grumpy, aggressive, and generally not someone you wanted to be around, lying about on a sun lounger all day, not interested in family life at all. On these holidays, I would take myself off for the best part of the day just to keep out of the way. My mother's focus would be on my sister anyway, so really it would have been a lot better if they had left me behind at home.

On this holiday, on about the third day, my father had disappeared and my mother asked me to go and look for him. I was somewhat reluctant to do this, knowing from previous so-called holidays what sort of condition he could be in by now. I found him propping up the bar, which was on the ground floor of these apartments. Fortunately, he didn't see me, but I could already hear he was extremely drunk. I will never forget the barman looking straight at me and gesturing to take my father out of his bar. I just looked back and shook my head, returning to my mother and sister, telling them the situation. My mother knew we'd never get him out of there – he never listened to anyone when he was miserable and sober, and he definitely didn't listen to anyone when he was drunk.

So here we were in a foreign country – a very unconfident mother with two children, having to walk to the nearest town to have the evening meal (probably about a mile or so). This was ok when we walked down in the evening sunlight, but I did feel that I had to be in control and take care of them both (my sister was only eleven). This surely wasn't a responsibility that should have been put on my head, even though I was, as the older generation would say, 'old for my years'.

After the meal, it was by now pitch black and my mother really didn't want to walk back in the dark, but she also wasn't too keen about getting into a taxi (a stranger's car). So again, I had to step up and get the taxi, and I got into the front seat. Even though I looked mature, I was very shy and unconfident. I was scared stiff sitting in a strange car with a driver who spoke hardly any English. I was struggling with English and French, let alone Spanish. I can remember jumping out of the car and getting the money from my mother and just stuffing it into the driver's hand, hoping it was enough.

It was time to head back to the apartment – gingerly, I will add. My father never picked on my sister, even paralytically drunk and raging like a mad bull, but it was a different story with me and my mother. As we walked down the corridor to the front door of the apartment, I could feel the anxiety building between us. To be honest, it was more fear on my behalf – I was fearful of him up to the age of fourteen, even when he was sober, but when he was drunk, that was another level. I was literally scared witless of him – my heart used to race at such a pace it felt like it would burst out of my chest.

As we got to the front door, I put my ear to it to see if I could hear anything (hopefully snoring), but there was nothing. *Oh, great,* I thought, *he's still in the bar – what sort of state must he be in now?* So my mother and sister went in to the apartment and I went down to the bar just to see what the situation was. Then the barman came over to me and started speaking loudly (you know how the Spanish seem loud to us, they seem to speak excitedly) which really upset me, and I just started to cry. I couldn't help it. When he saw the tears, he completely changed – he put his arm round my shoulder and in his best broken English told me that he and some of his friends had to escort my father out of the bar and as my father wouldn't tell them the apartment number and clearly didn't want to stop drinking, they had left him outside the building on the steps. Well, that was how I interpreted what he meant. The only thing that was absolutely clear was he kept saying, "Angry man, very angry man." I perfectly understood that in both ways, having been on the end of that anger on too many occasions.

But there was no sign of him. So my father was missing in a foreign country, paralytically drunk, and we were left in the apartment on our own. I did once more go out of the apartment block to see if I could find him, but I couldn't.

By about 11pm we were all in bed. This apartment only had

two bedrooms, and I had to share a twin bedroom with my sister, which was testing as it was, as we didn't get on very well. In the early hours, probably about between two and three o'clock in the morning, there was a huge bout of banging on the entrance door – it sounded like someone was trying to knock it down – accompanied by a load of shouting. I started shaking and my heart by was beating so fast I could hardly draw breath. Suddenly, my sister and I heard a load of crashing and glass breaking, shouting and swearing. My sister began crying, and I was trying to console her, but we were stuck in this room with bars up the windows – there wasn't any way out at all. I could hear my mother crying and then screaming as he threw her around the living area, and there was one point when it all went quiet, just for a few minutes, and I thought, *He's killed my mother.* Now you might be thinking, *If my father was seemingly trying to kill my mother, scared or not scared, I would go in and protect her from him!* But I didn't know what to do. I had my sister crying inconsolably and a fear of him like you would fear fighting a lion – the sheer hope that luck might go your way but really knowing that even if you do what seems right you will not get out of that situation alive. (That fear changed later, and if you keep reading, you will find out why.)

Then suddenly the silence broke and the crying and screaming started again. I can remember my mother shouting at him, "The children, the children!" This I think somehow did finally resonate, and after a further bit of commotion, things all went still.

When the dawn broke the following morning and my sister and I got up, gingerly opening the bedroom door, I could see my mother just sitting on the settee nursing a cup of tea and still shaking from what had happened. I looked around the apartment at what looked like a burglary or even a murder scene. There was smashed glass everywhere. The pictures that had been on the walls in the entrance were on the floor with the frames broken, the tables no more with glass all over the floor, and to make it even worse, there was blood all the way down the walls.

I spoke to my mother and asked where the blood had come from. She very slightly grinned (in a 'don't worry' kind of way) and said, "No, it's not mine, it's your father's." She said she didn't know what had happened, and obviously he wouldn't be able to fill in the blanks because he wouldn't have any memory of what had happened either, as per usual, but there was blood everywhere, over the floors as well as over the walls.

All the local barmen talked to each other, and we later found out from the original barman what had occurred that evening. He had left my father on the steps of the apartments, but my father had then staggered to a taxi and gone to the nearest town where all the bars were and went into the closest bar to carry on drinking. But after a number of drinks (and by now he was getting seriously aggressive), some of the local men in the bar had tried to take him on to throw him out into the street. But they quickly realised that, when he was drunk to that level, all he wanted to do was kill, and yes, when I say 'kill', I am not exaggerating (although I haven't concrete evidence). I'm pretty sure this had happened before when he was drunk. One of the locals hit him over the head with a bottle, and even this did not bring him down the first time, so they hit him again and finally managed to knock him unconscious and then throw him into the street. What we are not certain about that evening was how he got back to the apartments paralytically drunk and covered in blood, but he did (unfortunately).

Now, my mother being daft as a brush, then spent the next two days thoroughly cleaning the apartment while he slept the whole fiasco off. When he did rise, as usual, he said nothing – just walked around silently for about two to three days then was back to his usual grumpy, moaning self, having filed what had happened firmly in the back of his head. Along with a nasty cut.

I should just explain what sort of drunk my father was. He would not drink anything for say Monday, and Tuesday but by Wednesday, he would be really grumpy (more than usual), so he would go out that night and just keep drinking until he couldn't stand up anymore – not always, but more often than not. You see, his problem with drink was once he had started, he didn't have any willpower to stop until he would suddenly drop to the floor. In fact, the addiction to the alcohol was so strong, he could drink ten pints of lager then go into the cloakroom and be sick and then come back into the bar area and carry on drinking. I had seen him do this myself, which was no mean feat, even for a seasoned drinker, as I found out in later years.

After about six – seven pints, he would be swaying about and starting to argue over the pettiest things. It was at this point I knew how thing were going to progress, and it wasn't going to be good. He would progressively become more and more angry with everything and everyone and was basically spoiling for a fight. He would come out with things like his army stories, the 'good old days' when he was in the armed forces – totally abhorrent.. He would also talk to me (even at the tender age of nine and ten) about his sex life with my mother, in detail. Because he was such an aggressive man and I was frightened of him even more when he was drunk, I just had to stay still and listen. He would get so angry it was like he was spitting venom – he would tell me everyone was scum; the teachers, the doctors, the police, you name it. A selection of people were all scum who didn't know what they were doing, and he knew better. You couldn't come across a more arrogant man, and with drink inside him, it just inflamed his issues.

This sort of behaviour happened on any holiday we went on. I would rather not have had any holidays because really the term didn't fit – it was more like going on a nightmare.

The problem with anyone who drinks to excess is that they have hardly any memory of any trouble caused, be it verbal or physical, when they wake up after the event. But the people on the receiving end have these words and actions embedded in their memory. If things that have been said were hurtful or, as with my father, downright nasty, bitter, and twisted, the recipient has to deal with it. This is particularly difficult for a sensitive teenager and would really hinder the development of any child. It definitely did to me.

***

On one holiday, we got to know another family with a son and daughter who were similar ages to me and my sister. At the airport, I had seen a book that said on its cover, 'So you want to be a racing driver?' by James Hunt, so I ran over to it and bought it. If I remember correctly, my father asked to see the book, looked at it, then gave it to me and didn't say much, and my mother – well, no interest at all. As with most racing drivers, it was go-karting where James Hunt started.

Well, on this holiday, the other father (we'll call him Barry) suggested the boys went go-karting. Because I was thirteen, unfortunately I wasn't allowed on the bigger adult karts, so his son and I got stuck on these slow 'kiddie karts', but Barry wasn't happy about this and was of the character to say something, which he did. The Spanish owner said he was more than happy to let the bigger lad (that was me) in the adult kart "because of the way he's driving", but wasn't so keen to let my new friend on the same. To be honest, I don't think my new friend was that bothered anyway, but me, I loved it. And when I got into the bigger kart, it was out of this world. At that age, I had never driven anything apart from a lawn mower.

Now this is where parents differ. My father barely looked at me going round the track at all – he was only there because this Barry had insisted and was eager to have a go himself. When we were leaving the centre, Barry was trying to buy one of the bigger karts for his son and was negotiating a price for the kart and delivery, whilst my father was not seen for dust and was having a smoke next to the bus, eager to be getting back to the bar. When Barry said, "Don't you want one of these? Your boy was bloody brilliant out there!" my father said nothing and changed the subject as soon as he could. Now I know we are not meant to blame our parents for things they could have done but didn't, but in this case I think it is justified. You ask Lewis Hamilton where he would be today if it hadn't been for his father's interest, commitment, belief, and love for his son to help him the best he could.

When people say you have to be a parent to know how to be a parent, I totally disagree. You have to be a child to say what you consider was good, bad, or poor parenting. You should know – you were the recipient. That's why you hear people say, "I'm not bringing my children up the way my parents did." They are judging their own childhood. For me, having an arrogant, self-opinionated, moaning father was the norm. Dealing with him when he was sober was hard enough – no matter what I did, I was always in the wrong for something.

I have spoken to other people who have had similar fathers. Personally, I think it is more about the person than the environment. By that I mean, if you see your father doing something that you think was wrong, then surely you would not do it to your own children. This partly explains the psychology of my father. *His* father was a drunk and deprived the family of everything, including food and clothes, in the pursuit of drink My father had said to me on a number of occasions that, no matter what, we would not go without. Yes, that was the term: "Not go without"! He had got it into his head that as long as we had food on the table and clothes on our backs, he could do whatever he wanted to in respect of his drinking. (Come to that, whatever he wanted in the respect of *everything*, really – he never asked for any kind of permission to do anything – he just did whatever *he* wanted to do). But he had fooled himself with the belief that he was better than his own father – and this only benefitted one person (and that was him). Was he so different from his father really? He would have liked to think so. He only had total contempt for his own father, constantly saying he had held him back and he could have done so much more if things had been different. (Same here, as you'll see.)

So family life went on in the same old way – the arguments when my father was sober and the silences when my mother wouldn't speak to him for days on end. We had a small King Charles Cavalier spaniel called Monty (chosen and named Montgomery by my father, mainly because of the snob value – but he never walked him and hardly acknowledged him). I used to use Monty as an excuse to get out of the house, and I'd walk him miles and miles, and whilst walking, I would be dreaming of a better life but not really having any idea of how I was going to achieve this.

***

Up to this point, I thought the upper school was a better place than my previous school. But things were about to take a different turn.

I was always a physically confident young man, and this helped in the physical battles of the past two schools, but it suddenly caused me a few problems in the upper school, and not just with the fellow pupils but with a certain couple of teachers. What happened was a real insight for me into adult behaviour. We were just finishing a PE session in the gymnasium. Before the lesson, I had asked the head sports teacher to look after some money I had with me to purchase a bike after school – it was one hundred and fifty pounds (a lot of money in 1984). He said I could put it in the safe in his office.

Once the PE session was over, all the lads were on a bit of a high with the adrenalin flowing, and when we got back into the changing rooms, one of the lads got onto a parallel bar and started doing chin-ups. Then another lad joined in to see who could do the most. Suddenly, someone called out to me to join in the competition. Now, I'm not a competitive person at all; well, not against others. I am only competitive against myself – so I was not at all comfortable. I felt I was being goaded to perform in front of the other lads. And it didn't stop there.

Within a couple of minutes (quite how it happened I'm not sure), the competition was to be between me and the sports teacher.

This teacher used to strut around the grounds in the summer wearing the smallest of shorts with his chest pushed out to its maximum, like a little rooster – this man had a serious ego and everyone knew it. If there was something that would fire me up, it would be to get one over (so to speak) on a teacher. The teachers at my school were not very helpful and definitely not supportive, so I didn't, I guess, have a huge amount of time or respect for them, especially the cocky ones. So the battle commenced. I was right next to my sports teacher doing chin ups. And yes, I did in fact wipe the floor, to rapturous applause from all the other lads as the teacher slunk off.

After we all got changed, I held back for the rest of the lads to leave before going to the office to ask for my money back, only to find that that particular teacher had already left – and, according to the other sports teacher, he had taken my money with him!. Frantically, I ran through the school until I found him taking a detention class. I knocked on the door, but he seemed to be ignoring me, and this angered me. I barged into the class and demanded my money back. To my surprise, he said he hadn't seen any money! Well, that was it ... I forcefully squared up to him and said in my straightest voice, "Unless you want a repeat of the embarrassment of earlier, you'd better give me my money."

He obviously knew what I meant, so he reached into his pocket and gave me back the money, then laughed and said, "I was only kidding with you." I just looked at him, turned my back, and walk straight out of the classroom.

For the next two years in that school there was underlying resentment and dislike of me from this teacher, but it did teach me (pardon the pun) some valuable lessons for the future, both in the school environment and in the outside world. It was really a good lesson in the ego of the human male (it's a lot less evident in the female, at least from my experience). Although my father, the only other male close in my life, was extremely arrogant and pretentious, I didn't detect any vanity – his is something that I have studied over the years from my childhood. In a school environment, word spreads quickly, and soon I was being treated like a king for defeating a teacher. However, this didn't last for too long before the pupils moved on to something else.

CHAPTER 8

Leaving hell (school) and fighting back with the first kiss

By the time I left the upper school, I had established quite a good rapport with some of the teachers. In the year before leaving school, we were asked to speak with the careers teacher, who in this particular school was actually the drama teacher. But he wasn't really that interested in what any pupil wanted to do, and he was definitely not a positive adviser, as you are about to see.

During this time, I had been taking woodwork (which I did find very easy and had a good aptitude for) and technical drawing. At this time, I used to design houses and draw the plans for them – I would cycle around the local towns and villages, looking at the different house designs and taking photos to help escape reality, or at least school and home life. I had a copy of an old set of architectural drawings for a house so I could see how the architects would draw walls and other prominent features, so when I would start to put a design into a set of plans, it really did look like an architect had drawn them (except the wording, which at that point I couldn't understand).

One day, my woodwork teacher, who also taught technical drawing, was covering a lesson, and he told us to treat it as a free period. So I got my folder out of my bag with the house plans that I was drawing and started working on them – we were in the technical drawing room and I had a drawing board to hand, so it seemed like a good opportunity. This teacher came behind me and just stood there looking, then he asked me a couple of questions about the design. Just before we left the class, he asked me if I could hang on and speak with him – he said he had a friend who was an architect and he would love to show him my designs. Would that be ok? "Well, certainly," I said, with a small amount of excitement, I must admit.

A couple of weeks later, the same teacher told me his architect friend was very impressed and said I should without question pursue this as a future career. But when I went to the careers advice teacher, he just said to me, "What class are you in for English?" I told him I was in the B class (in other words, not the brainiest group), and then he said, "And maths?" I told him the same, and then he said "You haven't got a chance of ever being an architect in those classes – now, what else can you do?"

So I said, "I'm good a woodwork and art." With that information, he said, "Well, there you are – a carpenter! You don't need such high grades for that."

When I tried to tell my father, he agreed with the teacher and said, "It's not your fault you're not as brainy as me – you've got quite a bit of your mother in you."

Well … He was sober and this was one of the rare occasions when I did bite back and said, "If you're so brainy, how come you are only a carpenter yourself?" This did not go down well at all, and in fact within a few minutes, I had wished I'd done what I normally did and just stayed quiet, because I then got all the excuses why it was the whole of his family's fault that he hadn't got a better education and a better job. I had heard this all before. But what your parents tell you, whether as a child or a young adult, you believe. Aren't your mum and dad meant to be the most trusted people you will ever know?

It was a few years after this careers advice (ha! Ha!), after talking to an older acquaintance who was just finishing his apprenticeship and had a car that I had been dreaming of owning myself (he was an electrician) that I said to my father I'd changed my mind about training as a carpenter. I wanted to train as an electrician, and I asked if his friend (drinking buddy, actually) would give me an apprenticeship. My father just looked and me and said, "You can't be an electrician, you're not bright enough!" Followed by, "You see, James, the trades go in an order intelligence – the brightest are electricians, followed by plumbers and carpenters, then you have the painter and decorator and finally the thickest (his words, remember, not mine) are the plasterers who don't really need a brain at all." And like a fool, I believed him.

***

My father thought he knew the lot and had an answer for everything (except how to live without alcohol and smoking, which was something else he tried to give up without success).

Yet he would bully me mentally, not just when he was drunk but also when he was sober – telling me how bright and clever he was and how he was the strongest person I would ever know (mentally, that is). But until I was fourteen, he also thought he was the strongest person I would ever know physically.

He would 'play fight' (or so he called it) with me, but most of the time it seemed he was just trying to prove a point, that he was so much stronger than me. In these 'play fights', he would always get me into a position where I was having to beg for mercy, and even then he would sometimes just push that little bit more. This mentality I really didn't understand – he seemed to get pleasure out of hurting me, but physically, I was a very resilient child and young man, and I was growing stronger by the day. He would have my arms twisted up behind my back, asking me to give up and pushing until I had to give in to him, because everyone has a cut-off point. I really don't know just how far he would have gone if I had refused to submit at some stage.

When I was fourteen, he grabbed me for another one of those so-called play fights. But I thought, *No! This is not going the way it usually does.* As he was trying to get my arms twisted round my back, I lifted him right up above my chest and threw him on the sofa. I just stood looking at him lying there, and he just looked back at me. Suddenly, he got up and walked off, and we never had any more of those so-called play fights ever again.

At the time, I really wondered why my own father did not like me. What had I done? I know he and my mother said that I was a little terror when I was aged two and three, but I found out it was quite common for young children in their second year to play up and test their parents' patience. But both my parents seemed to carry this resentment through my later years as well. Perhaps the fact that I was a honeymoon baby (basically an accident) didn't help. I think resentment was at play here!

I think at this point in my life I was starting to be very mentally confused with my own behaviour and definitely that of others. To add to this confusion, I had met a girl at the high school – a year younger than me and about two inches taller! But I wasn't very good with the opposite sex, even though others thought I was. In fact, being shy was not something girls admired – they seemed to like the big mouths and the boys with attitude always looking for trouble. Those boys seemed to always get the best girls – the girls who you would give your right arm for a date with. This was something else that was confusing – why would a girl put up with being treated badly by a boy who thought more of himself than her? But time and time again, there it would be, the same scenario. As an adult, and after many years of observation and talking, I understand more than I did, but at fourteen, it was just something else in one's head to fathom.

As I said, I met this girl, and as with many initial meetings, it was her best friend that asked me to meet her. I saw her every day, any time we had free. And I had my first real kiss with her – and what a kiss! They say you never forget your first, and I never have.

Mentally, ignoring the home and school life, I was very mature for that age, which is why I found it very difficult to get on with any of my peers. Even my best friend and I had difficult times understanding each other sometimes. For example, for Christmas, when I was fourteen, I received my own electric razor, but my best mate got one of the first video games and was so excited by it. I would spend my time thinking about relationships and whether I would like to have children one day, and my best mate just wanted to play a game. Now you can see why I had so many problems fitting in anywhere ,because the people who I could resonate with were all ten years older than me and didn't want to be around a fourteen-year-old, which was totally understandable but didn't help me much.

But however mature I may have been, dating girls was still new to me. After a few months of dating, I found the amount of time she wanted to be with me was getting too much for me, as I wanted to work in the school holidays and not just sit with her. If I'm totally honest, the fact that she was two inches taller than me did bother me too! I know this may sound selfish, but I wasn't prepared for the intensity that she clearly wanted, so I called it a day with her, something that I regretted very soon after. She was very upset and wouldn't even speak to me. Unfortunately, she got in with a bad crowd shortly after our splitting up and got involved with drugs and other things she shouldn't have, and I felt a huge pounding of guilt for what had happened. I had tried to speak with her, but she wouldn't listen and instead just told me where to go. I felt this guilt, rightly or wrongly, for a number of years. As we were in a small town, you never lose track of what people are doing, and you can always find out. Oh, and just to add to my regret, a year later I was the same height as her and ended up being taller than her – adolescence, hey!

I had a few very short relationships after that but mainly just worked with my father and his brother in the building trade, which at that age I enjoyed. I enjoyed the physical side immensely, and I was always with adults and not children. On top of all that, I was getting money, something that clearly was a great motivator for me as I was learning what sort of person I was and was becoming. The downside was the fact that I was totally controlled by my father and was being even more saturated with bad attitudes, opinions, and beliefs, which would cause me some great problems later in life.

The year I became sixteen was just as difficult as the rest had been. Even at that age, I was having trouble with negative thinking and over-thinking – as the psychologists later called it, over-analysing. From time to time, and sometimes from moment to moment, I would have trouble thinking there was a future for myself. It just seemed so difficult and frightening – would I be able to achieve the things that I wanted? I knew how to work hard, but was that going to be enough? The other major thing that I would constantly feel and spend a lot of time thinking about and analysing were relationships. I can remember on many occasions walking the dog and going through scenarios of meeting new girlfriends and their parents and how I would want that to be – how I would want them to see me as a person. Then I would tell myself I was wasting my time because I wasn't really good enough for someone to feel about me the way I wanted them to, and the negative thoughts would start to creep into my mind. How would I ever get out of the family home and how would I cope on my own? At this point in my life, my father had made me completely dependent on him, yet I needed to get away from this man who (I know now, looking back) was destroying my mind and me as a person. At sixteen, I seemed to have a million things to think and worry about all running around in my mind, and sometimes it did feel very overwhelming, when really, at that age, the only worry I should have had was getting my homework in on time.

So here we are at the final year end of school (hooray!). As you have probably realised, school was not something I was going to miss. But would college be any better? At this point, I would not know until the end of summer. So what about home life? It carried on much the same – my father was still getting drunk two or three times a weekend; the rest of the time he was best avoided. My parents were constantly arguing or my mother wasn't speaking to him at all. And now my sister was slowly going off the rails.

But amidst all this going on, I had decided to start on my journey into weight training. When I was at the upper school, I joined the weight lifting club, which had the benefit of being able to use the local leisure centre facilities (weight room) and a fully equipped commercial gym, and it wasn't long before it was clearly something I was able to excel at.

The club was run by one of our sports teachers (another egotistic character). I also remember us all (the boys) in the club one day watching over this teacher doing a bench press, when suddenly one of the lads in the club said out loud to the teacher, "Is that all you can lift, sir?" his didn't go down well at all, and with a scouring (and somewhat reddish) face, he lifted himself up from the bench and invited the boy in question to demonstrate *his* prowess with the bench press (in fact, it actually was more of an order than a request, to be fair!). The boy declined straight away, but in doing so he just as quickly offered me to the bench to beat the teacher. Suddenly, all eyes were on me. I could see in the boys' eyes what they were thinking – is he going to take this challenge? And to be fair, most of the boys, although from my year, didn't know me at all. My best friend (well, only friend really) was with me, though, and even he was wondering what I was going to do with this situation.

I had no wish to beat the teacher at all but unfortunately the teacher started to goad me to the bench with comments like, "Well, James, do *you* think you can beat me?" I had quite a fractious relationship with most teachers, and this was enough to at least have a go and see if I could embarrass the egotistic sports teacher. So with a deep breath, I took the challenge and went to the bench, and as I looked at the discs on either side of this bar, sitting on the stands, I though, *Can I? Can I really lift the same amount as this full grown man in his thirties?* I lay on the bench, and the teacher in question helped me position my hand for the best possible result (he obviously didn't believe for one minute that I would or even could lift what he was lifting at the age of just sixteen, but that is exactly what I did, and in fact it didn't end there, as he was so incensed that I had out-lifted him, he suggested that we go for more weight. I was in a predicament because I had all the lads cheering and totally elated as to what I had achieved and all the focus on me, which made me very uncomfortable indeed, so we lifted again and again until the sessions time ran out and we had to leave the gym.

I knew I was strong from lifting objects on the building sites I would work on in my holidays and spare time, and I loved lifting say a wheel barrow full of bricks, and on the next visit to collect more, I would think to myself, how many more can I lift from the last time? I would keep increasing until the wheel barrow couldn't handle any more without falling over. During these little self competitions, I started watching the World's Strongest Man competitions on the television and thought, *That is something that I would be good at.*

I was sixteen years old and had a weight lifting set in my bedroom that I was constantly using, but I was very lean (though not skinny), and people would say to me on many occasions, "Boy, you need to put some weight on!" So with a huge heap of muscle magazines (next to the huge heap of car magazines), I read as much as I could on gaining muscle/weight and set myself a diet to gain some weight with training. This worked well because in less than a month I had gained more than one stone (7kg) in weight, something that my father had made a remark on but was clearly not to impressed by. Also at this time of constantly reading these magazines on training and building muscle, I was wondering whether *I* could become a bodybuilder, (like Arnold) but the food you had to eat for the bodybuilding career was very restrictive indeed, and although I was lean/very slim, I loved my food (and still do!), so I looked at the career of strongman and thought this would be more suitable for someone like myself.

But when I watched the strongman competitions on the television, they were all what I considered fat (and strong). I really had a problem with the amount of fat that it seemed was needed in those days to lift those phenomenal weights. I knew that gaining mass was a way of gaining strength, and all bodybuilders had to do this in order to get more muscle mass. I had an issue with that too! It was the gaining fat part that was the issue, and now I look back and can see that this was (what psychologists call) a learnt behaviour problem. I had learnt from watching my mother yoyo with her weight, with the term "I'm just cutting down for a bit!" used almost weekly. I had learned this behaviour from her, and as a result I never pursued what could have been a very rewarding career in something that I loved doing. So I guess what I'm saying here is: listen to what you are thinking and question it before you make any decisions based on it. Your thoughts could be false or need addressing (which can be done), and you too could have the life/job/career you always wanted.

CHAPTER 9

The sister and the woman

My sister was the favourite. You might think I'm feeling sorry for myself, and I used to as a child, but it didn't work then and definitely doesn't work as an adult. But as a brother at school, I would look out for her as I was her elder by two years. She did not appreciate this at all. I didn't follow her around, but just kept an ear to the ground, and if there was any sign she could be in trouble, I would do my best to stop it. I don't know why – I felt it was my duty, especially at school.

By the age of thirteen or fourteen, my sister had got the drinking bug (obviously from our father as our mother barely drank at all).

The first time I knew there was a problem was one day when I was riding around the town on my motorbike (not being of age to drive a car quite yet but yearning for as much freedom as possible, I had a motorbike for a year or so). I came round a junction with a corner shop, and to my shock, there was my sister with three others around the same age, all drunk out of their heads, lying on the path. So I stopped my bike and went over to get her home. Well, I tried to help her, but I was met with a torrent of abuse; swearing and so on. At the time I thought, *She's just like our father – oh, great that's just what the family needs.* She wasn't going to listen to me.

After the abuse she gave me, I was in two minds whether to

just leave her there lying outside the shop, but as usual, boring old bruv was going to do the right thing. So I got back on my bike and rode home. I told my mother (my father wasn't home – ironically, he was probably propping a bar up himself). My mother drove with me back into the town, and my sister and her friends were still sitting outside, even more drunk than when I had left them, two of them still holding onto what was by now an empty vodka bottle. We had to get her to the car and then home, where my mother looked after her.

I'm sure some of you may have started experimenting with alcohol at a young age, but drinking a whole bottle of vodka by yourself at thirteen? And it wasn't the first time she had done it, as it turns out. I also discovered she was smoking rolled tobacco that she was taking from my father and hiding in her room. She was very confrontational over nearly everything I spoke to her about, but as usual my mother made excuses for her behaviour, blaming it on her being a young teenager. I personally wasn't convinced, due to the abuse she had served me in the past when I was only looking out for her – I just thought, *You've got a bad attitude, just like your father.* If it wasn't bad enough having one drunk in the family, now it seemed we had two.

To make matters worse, when my father was told of this, he spoke to my sister, but obviously, being a drunk himself, he was very limited as to what he could say. What he could have said, had he not been such an arrogant man, was, "Look what it's done to me. I'm trapped by this and it's destroying the family and will destroy you if you let it, so let's sort this now before it gets out of hand." But instead, he said nothing of the kind. He could not admit the problems he had with the drink, or smoking, come to that. (I should just point out that I am not a hater of drinking or smoking or anything that brings some relief to someone's pain. Just as long as it doesn't bring pain and suffering to others in the process. These are just the experiences that I have had and my opinions on those experiences.)

**

For a while, my sister tried to keep away from trouble by staying in her room night after night, which wasn't a bad thing – at least I didn't have to worry about where she was. And my father didn't always come back and cause trouble – sometimes he would stagger home, drop on the settee, and just sleep, as long as he didn't encounter any person on his way to the settee.

But one Saturday night, he and my mother had been down to the local club (similar to a pub but voluntarily run for the village community), and as usual he was completely drunk. He decided to invite a few people back home afterwards, most of them as intoxicated as he was. So five men and a woman came back to our house. The woman (let's call her Rainey) was engaged to one of the men (Bill), but she had a reputation for being a flirt. She had come on to a few of the single men, only for them to be blown away when they acted on it. This was her way, and by now everyone knew it – to be honest, it still didn't stop some of them from trying again and again, but she was loyal to her fiancé, or so I thought …

There were five men in our kitchen shouting, laughing, and generally making a lot of noise, so I came down from my bedroom and went into the sitting room, only to find my mother looking worse for wear. This was unusual, and next to her on the settee was Rainey. I went and sat next to my mother, and even though I knew she favoured my sister over me, I still felt a huge sense of responsibility and protection for her. I asked her if she was alright, and she started to speak to me, saying she couldn't understand why she felt so bad.

While we were talking, Rainey to the other side of me was rubbing her hand up and down my thigh and sending a tingling up and down my body that I'd never experienced before, and I was rather enjoying it, to be honest. Then my mother then got up and said she was going to bed, and I followed her to the bottom of the stairs to make sure she was alright. I then turned round only to find Rainey standing right behind me, and before I could say a word, she pushed me into a room that my father used as an office, shut the door, and locked it. My heart was racing at such a rate I didn't know whether it was from excitement or fear. Within seconds, Rainey was all over me. She had her leg wrapped round me like a Boa constrictor getting ready for its breakfast, and her tongue was firmly navigating in my mouth. I'd thought my first kiss was a wow and special, but this was off the Richter scale … If this was what the adults were up to, it was wonderful.

I reckon the kissing and hugging only lasted a few minutes before someone was trying to get through the door and making quite a song and dance at the fact that it was locked. At this point, I knew the racing heart was definitely from fear – it was my father trying to get into his own office. As he was drunk, I reckon if we hadn't opened it when we did, he would have smashed it in. As the door opened and he fell through it, he never said a word about the fact that Rainey and I were locked in that room together. In fact, I don't think he even registered who we were. *What a relief* I thought as I started to walk upstairs. I was hardly aware of Rainey following me up, but on the landing, she suddenly planted herself right in front of me and said (looking straight into my eyes), "James, I love you, I really do love you."

I just replied, "Rainey, you're drunk – let's see if you still love me in two days." She protested then that she really did love me and wanted to be with me, and I said, "I'm sixteen – you're ten years older than me," but she said she wasn't bothered about the age difference if I wasn't.

Talk about emotions flying. As these words were being exchanged and Rainey was leading me to my bedroom, suddenly my mother came out of her room. She saw us both but just said, "Where is your Dad?" I told her I had just seen him downstairs, but she asked me to go and find him. As I walked with Rainey holding my hand very tightly down toward the kitchen, she started to show affection again, but at this point, the kitchen door opened, and I could see Rainey's fiancé looking right at me. Now my heart was racing again, and I was thinking, *Does he know? Has he any idea about what has been going on?* As I looked into the kitchen, suddenly there was a more pressing situation. Five drunken men and my father (by far the most dangerous) were looking at and swapping my father's gun collection. My father had a number of guns, all with ammunition. Now, you don't have to be Einstein to realise that loaded guns and drunken males are not a good combination. Now the fear was back, and my thought was: *How on earth am I going to get this situation sorted without someone getting hurt?*

So I used Rainey to try to break up the party, so to speak. I said, "We've got a real problem here – you need to take Bill home, and hopefully the others will go too." This partly worked, apart from one young man who didn't seem to have anywhere else to go. He was determined to remain with my father drinking, so I went off to try and get some sleep (yeah right). Well, that was a joke with the two in the kitchen below, but then it all seemed to quieten. So I crept down the stairs, and to my relief both the young man and my father were asleep on the sofas. With that, I unloaded the guns and went back to my room.

But sleep? No... I just couldn't get what had happened earlier with Rainey out of my mind. I kept asking myself *Could it be true? If I speak with her in a couple of days, will she remember?* And if she did, what then? Inside, I desperately wanted her to remember and leave her fiancé to be with me.

The following morning, I got up early and took the dog for a walk to try, I suppose, to clear my head. But instead, all I could think about was the 'what ifs'. My head was spinning with so many thoughts, emotions, and feelings that I was finding it hard to make any sort of sense of this. My normal senses of reasoning and logic seemed to be disappearing in a mist of willingness. The total willingness for this to all be right and true and for me to be with someone of an age that I could (strangely) get on with. In the next few hours, the fog in my mind was now getting so thick I could hardly breathe – all I could think about was Rainey every minute. I could not concentrate on anything at all, yet I felt trapped. This woman (not girl) had told me she wanted to be with me, that she loved me, and somehow, I needed to speak with her to find out if this was still the case when totally sober. These thoughts were completely screwing with my head.

Well, two days passed, and I had heard nothing. My mother would look at me, as if she knew something but didn't say anything – nobody, especially Rainey, was saying anything, and this was driving me mad. It was then I thought *Right, I'm going to have to ask her outright.* I needed to know but was scared to, in case the answer wasn't what I wanted.

So on the third day, my father was going to the club, and (unusually for me) I asked to go with him. As we walked in, I clocked Rainey sitting quietly in the corner, which wasn't like her at all. I just froze for a minute and tried to look the other way. But I couldn't take my eyes off her – my stomach was spinning and I really didn't know what to do for the best. I remember the confusion was immense, and I was nearly at the point of being physically sick when I decided to go to the gents' cloakroom. I really thought I might be sick, but I also hoped she might follow. Well, that's what she did. She walked right up to me, face to face, and I could hear myself say, "I bet you don't remember what happened the other night?" She leaned closer, so close I could hear her heart beating, and said, "Yes I do, James, and I still mean it."

Quickly, I retorted, "Mean what?"

She replied, "That I love you."

Just then, her fiancé came through the door! My heart was nearly going sideways when he looked at me and asked if I was alright. By the time I'd answered and turned round, Rainey had gone into the ladies, and I then went out the back door just to sit down and wonder, I suppose.

Rainey and I couldn't talk any more that day, and then I didn't see her for a number of days. This was driving me mad – literally. As you will all know, being in love or infatuated with someone is wonderful if it's reciprocated, but if it isn't, it's torture, especially to a sixteen-year-old. With everything else that had happened that year with the old man and my sister, I just felt I'd had enough. At sixteen, I'd had enough. So I took myself off walking. I just walked and walked and cried and screamed as well. When you're in a forest, nobody can hear you scream (wasn't that in a film?). The forest was my sanctuary. I felt safe and at peace there – it was a place where I could escape from reality, and boy, I needed to. It was where I could dream, gather my thoughts, and contemplate things. I would run there every time in times of trouble.

On this occasion, I'd been gone for a number of hours but finally decided to go home. When I got there, a strange thing happened (well, strange to me). My mother came to me and said, "I know about Rainey and what happened."

By then there was nothing else to say about that – I hadn't seen or heard from Rainey in over a week, and that said it all to me. I just looked at my mother and said, "Mum, I've had enough. I've had enough of everything, the whole lot, *everything*!"

You have read a fraction of the things I had been dealing with up to this point. For this book, I've had to pick the more relevant situations, but there were also things like having teenage spots over your face and needing to start shaving, which only made the spots worse,… When you are very shy and unconfident, the last thing you need is a face full of spots, and when all your peers judge on superficial things like looks, it really does become a major problem – I hated them and in turn hated everything about the way I looked, because of the restriction I felt they were putting on me, and nothing anyone could or did say would change those feelings. I wouldn't go out to meet anyone for weeks and sometimes months at a time. I would just walk the dog and dream – dream of finding a nice girl with a good family, preferably without any drunks in it; dream that one day my father would give up the booze and we would build up a family business, together with offices and workers. (That definitely was just a dream in both parts. Giving up the booze? Yeah, right. And the family business turned out to be a joke too.) And now there was this situation with Rainey.

Well, my mother, as usual, didn't know what to say or do. So she got my father to speak to me, who, with no compassion at all, told me that it was just a crush and I'd get over it. I can remember sitting outside on a log with him preaching over me and just looking up once and saying, "You really don't understand. I don't want to be here anymore," and then I shouted as I ran off, "I've had enough, it's over!" To this day, I don't know why, but after this outburst, my father for the first time in my life *asked* me to do something instead of ordering me, and that request was to go and get in the car. By then, I wasn't in the frame of mind to question anything, and I just got into the car, not knowing where we were going at all, until we got to the GP.

The strange thing was that I had this overwhelming desire to get out of it all, but I hadn't thought about how on earth was I going to do it, so perhaps it was just a cry for help. After shouting at my father, I just seemed to shut down and not want to say anything. I can remember feeling a bit distant from reality – it was very peculiar and un-nerving, but not frightening – very strange. My father told his version of why I felt the way I did (I wasn't in the room). Obviously, the family life didn't come into it at all – he would have blamed the whole lot on Rainey. I remember I just sat there outside this office thinking, *I've got to find a way out of here.* Then the doctor asked to speak with me alone, which my father was reluctant to do. I thought, *He's not bothered about me – he's bothered with what I might say about him.*

As it was, by then, I really couldn't have cared less what was going to happen. So the GP spoke to me and said, "I'll give you some tablets and you come back and see me in a month's time."

For some reason, I did react and said, "Don't bother because I won't be here." Well, with that, he called my father into the room, and the next minute I was being taken to the hospital, where I would get to speak with a psychiatrist.

Again, I answered his questions, but I didn't add anything else. Then he asked to just speak with my father. I wondered what lies my father was telling him, and I wasn't wrong, for when they had finished talking, the psychiatrist said, "I've prescribed you some tablets, and in a few days you will start to feel a bit better. In the meantime, listen to your father."

"Listen to my father!" What on earth had he told him? No doubt how wonderful a father he is. But to his credit, my father didn't let me out of his sight for the next few days. Looking back, I would like to think it was out of genuine love for a son. But it was probably more out of the guilt, or the questions that might have to be answered, or the stigma of having a son commit suicide – would people blame him?

CHAPTER 10

The last of the teens

The next few weeks were quite testing for me. I had in that time seen Rainey, and she would just smile with her head slightly tilted downwards. After a number of weeks had passed, the pain from my encounter with a 'real woman' started to dissipate and the fog was starting to clear. After coming back from the hospital, my father told me I'd get over Rainey and there were plenty more fish in the sea. Then he said I just needed to keep busy, and he would make sure I was too busy to think about her. As for the anti-depressants, he told me there was no way I needed them and he didn't know what the psychiatrist was thinking of, giving a sixteen-year-old these. I did take the tablets for a couple of weeks until he found out. And then I stopped. He was constantly reminding me what the psychiatrist had said and that was to "listen to your father" (like I had a choice at that time). As if he needed another excuse to claim he was. But he insisted that I didn't need tablets and told me that I wouldn't be taking them. He thought a person weak if they had to rely on tablets. Better to rely on alcohol and cigarettes!

All I had been doing in the meantime was working around the house so as not to bump into anyone. My father had an idea of opening a shop and was at this time extending the garage to accommodate it, and I was helping with that. This basically meant he told me what to do and sometimes how to do it, and I just did as I was told. For those weeks, it suited me, and I was earning (as he always told me, "You don't do things for nothing").

***

Around this time, a serious incident happened. One morning, after a night of unrest in the house because of my father's drunkenness, I came downstairs to the kitchen very early because I couldn't sleep any longer. My mother was already there nursing a cup of hot tea and very tearful. So I asked, "What's wrong?" As if I didn't know... but on this occasion, I had no idea what she was about to tell me.

The previous night, in his drunken rage, my father had gone to his office and loaded one of the two pistols he had and went back upstairs, threatening to "blow my mother's head off," pointing the pistol right in her face.

I just couldn't believe it. I knew when drunk he was more than a loose cannon, but this was on another level. So after making my mother another cup of tea, I went into my father's office, and there on the desk was the gun, still loaded. I unloaded it (I'd had to teach myself how to do this. I wasn't at all interested in guns, much to my father's disappointment, but he did bully me once to watch how the gun worked and how you loaded/ unloaded it. I had to fire it as well, just to pacify him. I think, really, he was hoping that if I had it in my hand and fired it, I would suddenly be more interested in them, but I wasn't.) I put the gun back into the safe in the wall and left the ammunition on the desk on purpose so he would know I knew the combination to the safe and that I knew what had happened that night. But as always, nothing was said ever again, and my mother didn't want me to take it any further.

On another occasion when he was drunk (to the point he could hardly stand), he was threatening to blow up the whole village from his garage with, as it turned out, nothing more than distress flares (but we didn't know at the time that that was all they were). So he was standing (only just) with these canisters in his hands, saying he was going to blow the whole godforsaken village off the face of the earth when my Nanna (his mother) stormed out and, straight to his face, said very sternly, "Dennis, what are you doing? Put that down and get inside the house!" To our astonishment, he did … He did exactly what she had told him; no arguing, nothing – he was like a little boy. (I learnt that no matter how drunk someone was, there could still be strong emotions associated with certain people (e.g., a parent), and past incidents or influences could be felt very strongly.)

***

It was nearly May of that year and I was coming up to being seventeen. I felt I'd been waiting for that year all my life. One afternoon when I was working on a site with my father and his brother, I saw a car for sale in a driveway – a bright blue Ford Escort. To cut a long story short, I bought that car, and once I'd got it home, still not having passed my test, I got the family car out of the garage and put my car in there. I'd frequently polish every nut, bolt, mud flap – everything. It was my first car, and at that point I loved it – it had done what it had needed to and taken over my life.

A few weeks after turning seventeen, I got my ticket to freedom and passed my driving test. I drove around for days and just kept filling it up – I loved it. I especially loved it when it was raining and I was completely dry and still moving, unlike when I had the motorbike. In fact, the rain and cold was one of the main reasons I went for a car instead of another bike (and it was a bugger getting intimate on the seat of a motorbike – enough said). So here I was – I had a car and money in my pocket (mainly for fuel). I still had the spot problem and a lack of confidence, but not with driving – in fact, I was probably a bit too confident on some occasions.

***

When my face (spot situation) allowed it, I would go to the skating centre four or five times a week where I had dated a number of girls, on and off. Around this time, I started dating a lovely girl a year younger than myself – dark-haired, tanned, and petite (we'll call her Susan). We seemed to be getting on really well, even though I had to stay away from home and work in London for several weeks at a time for a local advertising agency – creating sales offices with local themes (local to London that is) If anything, as the saying goes, 'absence makes the heart grow fonder'. One Sunday, everything seemed fine – I was due off on the Monday for the rest of the week. We said our goodbyes, and I said, "I'll see you at the end of the week." I worked in London up till Friday morning, putting in about 100 hours working round the clock to get the job done.

When I got home that Friday, I decided to go to the roller-skating centre because I knew she would be there. I didn't call her first – I thought, *It'll be a surprise*, and it was, but not the surprise that I was expecting. When she saw me, she wouldn't put her arms round me, and the kiss was very half-hearted, so straight away I said, "What's wrong?" to which I got the classic: "Nothing." Already thinking it was over, I went in with, "I've been working away all week like a slave, I get back at 5pm tonight, and really all I wanted to do was sleep, but instead I drag myself up here to see you, and what?"

She reluctantly admitted that she wanted to call it a day. And do you know the reason? "I'm sorry, James, you're too nice."

"Too nice?" I said. "How can someone be dumped for being too nice?" She didn't answer, but just walked off crying. *Well,* I thought, *that's a new one.*

A couple of months passed and I was in the town centre just coming out of a bar when I heard some commotion going on between a man and woman. When I glanced over to where the noise was coming from, I could see it was Susan, arguing with a bloke. Then suddenly he raised his hand and struck her on the side of the head, which knocked her briefly to the ground. I walked over, grabbed hold of him, had a word with him about hitting women, and then threw him over the wall that was behind us.

Susan got up and then she ran to me with her arms open. But I folded mine and said sarcastically, "No, no, no! Now I know what you mean about being too nice. Totally understand. Goodbye, Susan."

I started to leave when she shouted, "I know you still want me, otherwise you wouldn't have done what you just did."

But I just said, "I didn't do that for you – I did it because bullies like him shouldn't go round hitting women." And I walked off.

Another lesson in human behaviour, which although I definitely don't condone, not then and not now, is that some people just need to be slapped. It's strange to me because it's not what I believe, but there you go.

***

I may have been confident at driving my car, but I really wanted to improve my overall confidence. Although I was training regularly with weights and getting more into building my body, getting bigger and stronger wasn't making me more confident like it did for others. I thought, after speaking to a few people, that travel would do it, so I made my decision – I was going to go to the States and backpack my way around. So nine months after I bought my first car, I'd written out an advert for the sale of it, which, with some savings, was going to fund this trip. I thought I would have one last night at my local roller-skating centre as a goodbye ... Oh, how that night was going to change things!

After my experiences of dating so far, I had come to the conclusion that I needed a girl older than me, because even at seventeen, the young men my age still had the ability to act like five-year-olds and the girls my own age (even though they are meant to be more mature than their male counterparts) I found too juvenile as well. The girls I kept dating just seemed too demanding and too up themselves. So I thought, *when I get to the States, it's going to be older and more down to earth; straight talking* – not the prima donnas I'd been dating.

At the roller-skating centre, I met up with my old school friend who was with some others that I previously had avoided. Yes, I was judging books by their covers, but this night, knowing I was going to be on a plane by the time my money for my car was in the bank, I thought, *Well, it can't do any harm,* so I sat down with them. On the seat next to me was a girl that I had heard a bit about, from my best mate mainly – heavily made up with a short skirt and hair in shades of different colours; not my cup of tea at all. But since it was my last night in the UK and all that, we got chatting and got on really well – in fact, it was nice to speak to a girl (woman) who was straight-talking, not constantly searching for compliments and more interested in herself than anyone else. This girl (her name was Maria) was the complete opposite of that, asking me questions and very reluctant to speak about herself. What a breath of fresh air! I asked if she would like to go out some time just for a drink, and she said she would, so that was that.

It turned out that she already had a boyfriend who was in the army, but she told me after our first date that she had spoken to him and finished the relationship. She said it had started to die after he'd joined the forces. So we continued with this relationship, and the trip to the States was cancelled, at least for the time being.

During my time with Maria, there were problems along the way. Maria's stepfather seemed to think it was ok to beat her mother black and blue on a fortnightly basis, and if Maria got in the middle to protect her mum, he would hit her too. So I had to get her out of that environment. So after we got engaged, which was only a year after I had met her, I found a room in a house for women only that she could rent to stop any further altercation. The last thing I wanted was to get in a fight with her stepfather and end up in prison. But things with her, especially after getting engaged, did get a little bit more awkward. There was one occasion when we had a bust up and, if I didn't stop, Maria threatened to jump out of my car by opening the door as we were going along the dual carriage way. When I did stop, she leapt out of the car and ran across the carriage way and sat down in the overtaking lane. Luckily, she wasn't a big girl and didn't weigh too much for me to run across and lift her back to safety in the car, then she just broke down sobbing, saying how sorry she was, and then we carried on. Sometimes it was a tempestuous relationship and very difficult, but I did love her and really just wanted to help her, but I must admit, she didn't make it easy sometimes.

The relationship that started off as a breath of fresh air was quite often now full of tainted air, but it was my first serious relationship. Though my family was just as bad as hers, just in different ways.

It wasn't long before my sister was starting to play up again, going out more often and coming back later and later. And then there was the weekend from hell – a serious incident that yet again I had to deal with myself, even though I was still only seventeen.

My parents had gone away for the weekend, so little sis asked me if I could drop her and her best friend in town. (I may have been a boring old brother, but sometimes that suited her). They wanted to go quite early – about 4pm – but she had her reasons. I knew not to push the 'big brother' thing too much, unless it really was required, so I didn't ask any questions – I just dropped them both right outside Rollerbury (the name of the skating centre we used to socialize in). The mistake I made in hindsight was I didn't watch them go in. They both waved me off, and I went into the town to see if there were any of my mates floating about. After that, I was off to pick up my Nanna – she was staying for the weekend to keep eye on us – well, mostly my sister. It's pretty ironic that she was supposed to be looking after us, but I had to pick her up, as she couldn't drive!

As you might remember, my Nanna and I were extremely close, so when I got to hers, we had a cuppa before we drove back to our house. I asked her if she minded going back through the town as I wanted to see if any of my mates was about, to which she replied, "If you're happy, darling, driving around with your Nanna in the car!" (Bless her.)

"Doesn't bother me, Nanna, I'm not ashamed of you," I said.

We drove around, and the mate in question wasn't about, so we then started to head toward home. But something (I don't know what – fate? Karma?) made me drive past Rollerbury instead of the quickest route. I passed the car park and could see a huge crowd in there, including one of my best mates. Obviously, something was going on, so I quickly indicated and pulled in.

Leaving my Nanna in the car, I walked over towards my mate, not having any idea what was going on or what I was going to find. He was kneeling down on the ground and seemed to be holding something, and there were probably more than a dozen people gathered in a circle looking down. He saw me walking over and said, "Sorry, mate, I just found her like this!" It was my sister he was holding, totally unconscious, covered in mud and sick, and her clothes all torn. Honestly, my first thought was, *My god, has she been raped?*

I knelt down and tried to make my sister hear my voice, but she was completely out of it. But I could see she was still breathing. So I picked her up and went to my car, and my friend helped me put her on the back seat. Then my Nanna started asking questions, and I snapped at her, "Nanna, not now, just not now." I felt bad about that later, but she wasn't really helping at that point. My sister's friend was also slumped against another car – she wasn't able to stand up on her own, but at least she was conscious, unlike my sister. I lifted her into my car too and headed off home.

I had to pass the estate that the other girl lived on, and as we were getting closer, she started to cry and make a loud fuss about how she didn't want to go home – well, I bet she didn't as she knew how much trouble she was likely to be in. But I had to get my sister home first anyway. So I looked at her in the back of my car and said, "You're not going home yet, now shut up!" I admit, I was angry with both of them – how could they be so stupid? But I had to (again) sort the situation we were all now in, and getting my sister home first was priority, not her silly friend. But once I pulled onto our drive, the friend leapt out and tried to run (unsuccessfully, still being intoxicated). She got to the main road before I got a hold of her and pushed back into the car. By now, my Nanna had got out. I grappled with my sister who had already been sick once in the back of my car and was now vomiting again over me. My Nanna unlocked our front door, but I also told her to lock the other girl in the car. My Nanna, knowing what mood I was now in, didn't say a word (not that I would have hurt her for the world) – she just quickly went to the car and locked it as the girl protested vehemently at the window. I then shouted for my Nanna to come up the stairs and bring a bowl. I laid my sister on the bed and put her on her side (just using logic, as I didn't at that stage know anything about first aid) and said to my Nanna, "Stay with her, keep her on her side, and don't leave her. I'll be back as soon as possible."

She said, "Are you taking the friend home?"

I replied, "*Ohhh* yes."

When I went downstairs to my car, the friend said she needed the toilet, so I helped her inside and left her in there for a few minutes. But when I told her it was time to go, she wouldn't come out, so through the door I told her in no uncertain terms, "You either unlock the door and come out on your own or I'll kick the door in and drag you out." That did the trick.

Whilst driving her home, she was first pretty offensive, then she went the other way and was crying till we got to her home. She was trying everything to stop me taking her home, including coming on to me, but I was angry and just needed to get her home and let her parents know the state she was in.

When we got there, emotions were running high with her parents. It was midnight and pitch dark, and here I was, a complete stranger, banging on the door with their drunken fifteen year old daughter But eventually, while her mother helped her upstairs, I told her father everything that I knew. As I was telling him, he started to cry. Now this I did find strange and didn't understand at all. You see, the only time I saw any emotion from my father was when he was drunk, and the only emotion he showed sober was anger and misery. I'd not had, at that time in my life, enough experiences with grown males to see them showing emotions. This was completely alien to me.

As the father was crying, he kept saying, "I just don't understand," and I can remember thinking at the time, *Well, mate, if you don't understand what's going on, I haven't got a hope.*

I returned to home and went straight up to my sister's bedroom to relieve my Nanna, but instead we just sat there, both of us talking, keeping eye on her and watching her finally sleep.

The next day, as the sun rose, I went outside to inspect what once was my lovely clean car only to find dried sick everywhere, back and front, on the floor, even on the parcel shelf. I opened all the doors and just sat on the front doorstep of the house and looked at the mess. Then my Nanna came up behind me and sat down with a cup of tea and said, "We'll clean it up, it'll be as good as new." And together we spent about five hours cleaning up the mess in between checking on my sister. By now, she was very hungover, non-remorseful, ungrateful, and arrogant, and that's putting it mildly. Even though she should have been clearly out of danger, I didn't feel it was right to leave her in the house, plus, if I'm totally honest, I didn't trust her on her own. So I stayed in the house the rest of the weekend until my parents returned.

Just before they were to return, we had a row. She didn't want me to say anything to our parents, but I had to tell them. What's more, I was going to keep my Nanna there while I did as the only witness, otherwise they wouldn't take my word for it over my sister. She will always be the 'golden child'. When they got back and had settled down, I got all of us (apart from my sister who didn't want to be there) round the table. My parents sat there in disbelief when I told them. I remember my father kept looking at my Nanna as if to say, *Is he telling the truth?* No thanks for looking after the golden child, no thanks for sorting all the problems out with the other parents, no thanks for not calling them on the Friday night when it all occurred – no, no thanks at all. I'd had to sort it all out at just 17 years old.

And my sister never thanked me for stepping into her life (not even years later) and stopping her from making the wrong decision. Like when she got involved with the local drugs gang, still when she was only fifteen. I found out that she was dating one of the dealers, and I thought I need to nip this in the bud – drinking, smoking, and now drugs. *No... not if I can help it.* So I decided to step in whatever the consequences. I set up a meeting with this man in the roller-skating centre's men's cloakroom. He wasn't very good on the skates at all, so I did have that advantage because I was pretty ok on mine. I introduced myself and told him he was going to finish with my sister *now* and then leave (the skating centre), and he was not to say a word about this request, or else. He must have found me enough of a threat, because eventually, he did. I knew he had done it because my sister came up to me to give me her thoughts, or rather a slap, for yet again sticking my nose in, and I was told in very blunt terms to keep out of her life from now on. But on the positive side, I had got rid of the druggy. But I still had to pay him some money to stay away from her.

CHAPTER 11

Drunken males

You'll remember I said I was scared of my father when he was drunk (well, petrified would be a more accurate description) and I said that this did change somewhat later on. Well, now I'm going to tell you what made that psychology change.

It was one summer evening, and I was out driving with Maria when we decided to go and get some take-away fried chicken. I was in there for no more than ten minutes, and when I got back in the car, Maria looked like she'd been crying, which was strange because she'd seemed perfectly happy when I'd left her 20 minutes ago. She wouldn't tell me what was the matter, but as I was looking at her, I just saw her look over my shoulder, and as I turned my head, I could see this group of youths standing, drinking lager, and smiling. She saw me looking but said, "Leave it … Please … just leave it."

I was about to turn the key to the car when the one who obviously had the biggest mouth shouted something and then started insulting Maria – right in front of me. Well, what was I to do? I had taken on boys in school, but this seemed different – this felt like taking on three men. To add to the mix, they were all clearly drunk. Now what other drunk did I know who I was scared of? Oh, yes – my father. All these thoughts ran through my mind in probably twenty seconds, and the decision was made. (Now I know the right thing would have been to just

121

walk away, but I was young, and I was also, as I've said many times before, physically very confident, and I was very angry.) After a bit more abuse was thrown my way, I got out of the car and fronted the main man, who took a swipe at me.

I couldn't believe what had just happened – his fist came toward my face so slowly, if I hadn't moved and had thought a bit quicker, I could have caught it. So the second time he tried, that's exactly what I did – I grabbed his arm and twisted round until he fell on the floor. By then, the other two were coming toward me, and with my newfound knowledge, I just turned and said to them, "Come on, then." They both ran at me and ended up lying on the ground with hardly any help from me.

So that was an important lesson –99% of drunken people (not just males) are so slow in their actions when drunk, they are often not as much of a threat as you might think. It's all in the mouth, which seems to be the strongest and definitely the loudest organ, but they have nothing to back it up with.

This new information helped on a number of occasions when I was out dating in a pub or a bar and there was a male who was worse for wear and getting loud and aggressive. I would know that if the worst came to the worst, I was going to be fine. Unfortunately, this was not the case with my father – because of the sheer anger he had when he was drunk, he seemed to get stronger. I think what happened with him was that my bravery came as I got older and started to find my own identity.

By the time I could drive and had my own car, I really felt I had a bit more freedom. But with this freedom, I did feel that I was starting to find who I was as a person instead of being, as someone said once, a little version of my father.

They said, "Don't you have a mind of your own?" And they were right, I didn't. I wasn't allowed a mind of my own – I was told what to do and what to think because what he said was always right. I think because I have a certain number of my mother's genes in me, and my mother is on the whole a passive person (just with an almighty stubborn streak in her), I had the right temperament to be manipulated by a very domineering father. I never in those younger years argued with him – I think the first argument I had with him was when I was in my thirties. When I was younger, I wouldn't have dared to argue. I used to think I was afraid to argue, but now I think he actually made me *believe* it was wrong to argue with him. That is one of the main problems in people who suffer with mental health issues – their beliefs. For example, it was my belief that it was the alcohol that was the problem, because it couldn't be my father; he was the king of kings and knew everything (or thought he did) – the man who was never wrong! But later on, I understood it was the person that was the issue, not the alcohol at all.

***

One particular Friday, my father was down the club as usual and my sister was out in the local town (getting drunk, and still only fifteen). I had agreed to pick my sister up (who's the mug, I know), so I was sitting up late with my mother when we could hear someone trying to get the back door open. It couldn't be my father because it had only just turned eleven and he wouldn't be back until the early hours. I decided to see what was going on. When I opened the door, to my complete shock, it *was* my father, who swung through the doorway like a drunken ape, spitting and shouting at the same time. I knew better than to try to tackle him or ask what was going on. But my mother seemed to have other ideas (and at the time, I' wished she'd shared them with me first, but she didn't). She asked him what the matter was. She should have known that this would just make him worse.

Well, that was it – he was seething again with hatred, but this time it was towards a young lad (someone I was quite friendly with – let's call him Alec). I've no idea what Alec had done to make my father so angry, but he wanted to kill this boy, and he was riffling (pardon the pun) through the drawers of his desk, looking for something, when my mother asked what he was looking for (*Did you have to, Mum?* I thought). I was worried that if we both tried to speak to him, he might get a bit confused and try to kill my mother or me.

"*Bullets!*" he shouted, "*Bloody bullets!* I know they're in here." He had a safe behind a picture. Being drunk, he was having trouble with the combination, but somehow, suddenly it opened. He then took a pistol out with its ammunition and then loaded the gun.

He also had a gun cabinet where he kept shotguns that were licensed, but also a black thing called a riot gun that was able to fire seven cartridges consecutively. This one definitely wasn't licensed. He started to load this, and now we had a huge problem.

My mother was frantic with fear, but for the first time, not for herself, but for whoever else he was going after. "How on earth are we going to stop him?" she whispered in my ear as he headed out the front door. But I knew we couldn't. Becoming hysterical, she said, "James, he's got loaded guns, he's going to kill someone!"

I felt very calm, and said, "Mum, enough is enough – pack a bag and I'll go and get some things." My mother was completely bemused with what I was saying and doing, so I explained, "This is it, Mum – it's gone too far this time. Get some clothes, we'll go into the town to find Julia (my sister) and go straight to the police, and it will all be over." But she was still worried about my father killing Alec. I thought if we called the police, we could let them sort that out – with the illegal guns (as the pistols came from the Falkland's war in the 80s), he would be banged up for years, out of harm's way. But she said no.

I asked, well shouted, actually, "Why are you protecting him? He put a loaded gun to your head once when he was drunk and you're protecting him – *why*?" She didn't or wouldn't say, but later, she told me that at some point in their relationship, he had threatened, "If you ever leave me, I will kill your family." When I found out, I remember thinking, *Who do you think you are? Rambo?* Yes, if he was drunk enough, I really think he could and would kill them. But being that drunk, oddly, he had the ability to load a gun, but he was useless at driving whilst under the influence – when he did drive, he would usually get the vehicle stuck somewhere trying to cross a field. In reality, I don't think he could have got to her family, let alone killed them, but that kept my mother with him and also trapped me until I was old enough to move out.

After all that drama, for the record, he didn't kill anyone that night. I was so tense, worried, and frustrated. I'd reached a point where I almost couldn't have cared less what he did, and at least if my father did this, it would bring things to a conclusion of sorts and all of this would be over. So I didn't call the police. I decided I didn't want the responsibility for what he would do. But I *could* look after my mother and my sister, so I persuaded Mum somehow to get in the car. My father was so drunk, he hardly noticed us leaving. We left him in the drive and went and picked my sister up, worse for wear again, and when we got home, he was in the sitting room with a bottle of whisky. My mother and I left him there and crept off to bed, but I think my sister joined him.

I seemed to be always sorting problems out and not solving many, all down to belligerence and arrogance, mainly from my sister and father.

The one thing my mother and I did have in common was the fact that she wasn't a drinker at all. On Friday nights, my father would usually go to the club on his own. When he was out, my mother would sit on the sofa and read the local paper after watching the soap operas, normally munching on a Mars bar as a treat. Don't get me wrong – she would have a drink just to be social, but she really wasn't that bothered, and I had decided that I was going to be teetotal. My theory from the age of twelve was if I didn't start, I wouldn't have to endure the pain of trying to stop. Also, I didn't want to put any family that I might have through the misery that my father put me and my mother through. I'd seen my father on a number of occasions try to stop drinking, but he never could, so my logic was: *Don't start something you can't stop.* Simple.

CHAPTER 12

Relationships

My next big hurdle was my relationship with my then fiancée (Maria), which, due to her family, was always a bit troublesome. And here we went again – another test to my mental capacity.

It was the summer of '89 (not '69 as the song goes). I was nineteen and we were buying our first property together as I'd been desperate to get onto the property ladder and get out of the family home at last. When we moved in, things seemed to be turning in the right direction. I had a huge mortgage to pay, but I also had gone self-employed as a carpenter and builder with my cousin (seven years older than me). We had plenty of work as I had taken on many of my father's old customers. My fiancée was making a home out of the property we had bought together, which was nice to see. Just before Christmas of that year, we were invited to her work's Christmas do, and something peculiar happened that altered everything.

We were in this hall with the music turned up loud and most people up and dancing (apart from most of the men, who were propping up the bar as usual at these occasions). I went to the gents', and on returning to the main hall, I looked across the dance floor for Maria. I suddenly clocked her dancing with a tall skinny chap who can't have been much older than sixteen. As she was dancing with him, he was groping her, with his hand firmly on both cheeks of her backside. I made my way over to them, and as I got right beside them, I think he was having such a good time he didn't even notice me standing there. But the more disconcerting part was I don't think my fiancée was bothered by his behaviour. But I was.

I got hold of him and dragged him across the dance floor to the set of French doors at the end and threw him out of them (I did open them first, I might add). Generally, I'm not an aggressive person, but if the right buttons are pushed and there are principles that I feel need addressing, then I can be (or rather I could be) physically persuasive. As he went out of the doors and fell to the floor, I picked him up and put him against the wall, asking, "Well? Do you want to explain?" Suddenly, he went to lunge at me, but I restrained him and put him back against the wall. Then to my surprise, my fiancée came through the doorway, screaming at me to leave him alone, and stood between me and him.

Very quickly I thought, *Hang on, this is completely round the wrong way round.* I hadn't beaten *him* to a pulp – in fact, I had hardly touched him. So I pointed to him and told him not to move unless he really wanted to fight me. As I was saying this, I could see her looking at him with a look she shouldn't have had. Hand in hand (and not romantically), I took her back to the car and drove us home in silence, which wasn't a bad thing. (I was used to it with my mother, because on one occasion, she never spoke to me for a number of weeks until I broke the silence.)

When we got back to our home and I asked Maria what was going on, at first, she denied anything had happened and claimed I was just looking for trouble. (That couldn't have been farther from the truth – even at 19 years old, I'd had enough trouble to last the rest of my life.)

I obviously knew Maria well – we'd be dating for just over three years. I knew she had a temper on her (she had punched me in the face once during a heated argument). But what happened next completely threw me. By now we were shouting at each other, and it was a full-blown row. All of a sudden, she walked into the kitchen and returned with a knife in her hand, and we just stood looking at each other. I said, "Woooooo … what the hell are you doing? Put the knife down." I didn't shout, just said it calmly, but it didn't work. This calmness seemed to be like fuel on a bonfire – she went crazy and came straight at me with the knife.

Back when my father used to 'play fight' with me, he taught me what he had learnt in the forces about unarmed combat, including protecting yourself from a knife attack. Boy, that was relevant now.

I managed to grab the knife from her and throw it into the lounge behind me, then she came at me, punching and kicking like she was possessed. I got hold of her and managed to get her to the ground, then I got on top of her and wrapped my legs over hers so she could no longer kick and held her arms out to the side. But still she was shouting and swearing at the top of her voice, and it didn't seem to matter what I said or did – nothing was stopping her. For a moment, I stepped into a dark place as I moved my hand from her arms to her throat and had a firm grip. With both hands now firmly round her throat, she quietened, and then it was like someone switched a light on, metaphorically speaking – I suddenly let go and got up. When she leapt up to continue, I ran out of our home and got in the car. She was right behind me, hitting and screaming, shouting, "You're not going anywhere!" Suddenly, she took her shoe off and started to smash the windows in a bid to stop me driving off. As I screeched off the drive, she shouted, "I'll kill myself if you don't come back!" There wasn't any way on this planet I was going back, no matter what she said. I just thought, *You can't drag me into this now.* This was the last straw – I couldn't take the responsibility anymore. (People who shout things in anger don't normally follow through, anyway.)

I had no idea of what to do or where to go. First I thought I would go to my Nanna's, but I didn't really want to involve her as she wasn't getting any younger. So I decided to go back to my parents.

When I got there, they already knew what was going on, or rather Maria's version. She had been phoning every five minutes to talk to me. The phone rang before I could say anything, and my father said, "You answer it – she doesn't want to speak to us." But all I got from Maria was, "I can't live without you – come back."

I told her, "No, it's over – tonight was the final straw," and hung up, but it rang again and again and again and just kept ringing. I apologized to my parents and took the phone off the hook. I told my parents what had happened that evening and then said I needed some air. I walked down the village street in the early hours, just going over things in my head.

On my return to the house, all the lights were on and my mother came running out on the drive saying, "She's done it – she's taken an overdose!" I could feel the blood draining from my body, but I thought, *Here we go again, more silly games.* But no … as it transpired, my mother had re-connected the phone after I'd gone out, and my now ex-fiancée called and said she had taken all the paracetamol and vodka in the house and left a message that she wouldn't bother me anymore. My mother then called for an ambulance and the police went to the house. They broke in and found my ex unconscious with the empty vodka bottle next to her. They rushed her to hospital, pumped her stomach, and saved her life.

***

Once she was out of hospital and had gone and spoke to a solicitor, the fun started. I'll cut this part short because, apart from the stress she was giving me and her solicitor, it's not so relevant as other incidents. At this time of the acrimonious split, I found I wasn't feeling my normal strong self (physically) and was showing a huge loss of strength – my weight was dropping and I had a very sore and swollen throat. On a visit to the doctors, I was diagnosed with glandular fever, and it was literally draining the life out of me.

So I wasn't working, nobody was paying the mortgage, and nobody was living in the house either – what a mess. And that year (1990), the housing market crashed. So that meant, with an interest rate at 15.5% and a house worth £25,000 less than what we paid for four months previously, the option to sell was not on the table. But just to get to an end, I said, "Take everything out of the house, just have it." And with her family in tow, she did – even the light fittings, Toilet seat, and switches. What a bunch!

At this time, the house really wasn't my priority. I needed to get healthy and get back to work – had there been some work to get back to which there wasn't. So I was left with the whole mortgage to pay, very little work, and a stripped house that I couldn't rent out because I needed to have things like a cooker, carpet, etc, all of which had gone.

***

In those times (and believe me, they were a struggle), all I had was my training gear. A friend took the house off my hands by living in it and paying half the mortgage for me, which released me from that financial burden. After the glandular virus had cleared, I could concentrate on getting my health and fitness back, or rather, getting my body back, as I didn't have much in my life anymore (and definitely wasn't interested in dating). I threw myself into body building and joined a commercial gym with my cousin.

This cousin was also my training partner and used to train with me at my home gym, but we had outgrown this facility now and needed to be in a commercial environment. Soon there proved to be another one of those psychological learning experiences, which, since my time dealing with depression at sixteen, were now of great interest to me. As the training was increasing, and my shape and size increasing too, I was asking more questions on the hows and whys of the training principles from the owner of the gym, who himself was a professional bodybuilder and a Mr UK winner.

I began to develop an interesting theory around this time. I noticed that my training partner and cousin, who at school was in the lowest class ,whereas I was in the class second from the top, had a pain threshold a lot higher than mine. I started to wonder whether people with a high IQ have a lower pain threshold. I had a conversation with a GP who also trained in the same gym, and he could see where I was coming from, but he said he wasn't aware at the time whether there had been any studies to show that this is the case. I think so from my experiences, but it would be interesting to know if it is factual.

Anyway, after probably two years of hard training, I quit the commercial gym. The reason was this. One evening after a training session, the owner asked me to hang around to discuss training, as he had done on numerous occasions before, and I thought, *Here we go – now what am I going to have to cut out or increase? Hope it's not more tuna.* (At this point, I was getting sick of the sight of tuna, even in the tin.) But no, it wasn't about my diet at all. The next stage was to start injecting myself (yep, steroids).

I said categorically, "NO, that's cheating." But I was told every professional bodybuilder in the world is on steroids, all of them, without question. I didn't believe it, but he asked who my favourite bodybuilder was, and I said, "Well, Arnold, simple!" He said even the great Arnold Schwarzenegger was on steroids. This I really didn't want to hear because, since I was a boy of fourteen, getting my first barbell set and grabbing that muscle mag off the shelf with Arnie on the front cover, I'd read everything he had ever written and a whole lot more. There was no Google then, so I couldn't see if what he was telling me was right, but of course we all know now that he was right. I was gutted. So I just trained at home as and when I felt like it.

Besides, around this time, I had met a woman called Elizabeth through a mutual friend and was dating her quite seriously.

CHAPTER 13

Marriage (that's all)

For the past fifteen months or so, Elizabeth and I had been together every evening and every weekend. We had discussed children, and she told me she would like a big family – I remember that conversation like it was yesterday. I said I definitely wanted two, but "we'll see how we go". Even at the age of 12, I can remember saying to my Nanna I wanted two girls, that's all, and really this hadn't changed.

I also remember discussing how I wanted to design and build a house, just to see what the reaction was to this prospect. Elizabeth actually seemed excited by the idea and even asked me if that had always been a dream of mine. I said I'd rather someone else build it – it was the design part that I had been dreaming of since I was a boy doing those drawings. But the other huge factor was that, after my very short property experience, I really wanted to get rid of that mortgage as soon as I could, and I was more than willing to work as hard as it would take to do this. Elizabeth seemed interested, asking what sort of design I was thinking of, etc.. It seemed everyone who met her liked her.

One evening, driving her car to take her home, we were going down this country road when, coming up the T junction, I started to brake but nothing was happening. So I braked harder and harder, and still nothing, until my foot was on the floor and we weren't slowing at all. Thinking quickly, I decided, as I couldn't stop and I could see some lights coming, instead of just rolling in front of a car, I would speed up and get across before it got to us. Unfortunately, it was hard to determine the speed of the other car, and it was actually speeding – in fact, he was doing more than 80 miles an hour and hit our passenger side. At that speed, it flipped our car up in the air so high that it went over the fence on the corner field and landed the right way up without any glass at all and both doors completely crushed in. When it came to rest, I found myself just sitting still at the wheel that I had been holding onto for dear life, but Elizabeth was missing. I climbed out of the car over the bonnet and over the fence to the corner piece of grass, only to find her lying on the side of the road semi-conscious, not knowing where she was or what had happened. But in those few minutes before finding her, and then seeing her lying there without any movement, the feelings I had told me enough. Once we had recovered, I asked her to marry me.

So I was twenty-three and getting married. . I wanted to live in the property I still owned from the previous fiancée for a year or so before tying the knot. But Elizabeth wanted a big white wedding, and since we were in the deepest recession this country had ever seen at that point, and I was lucky if I worked one week in four, and even then it was for a significant rate cut, we could not afford a big lavish wedding. Then her father stepped up and said we could have the big white wedding and he would foot the bill … on the condition that we got married *before* we moved into my property. I'd already been through the fiasco of living with someone, but I took (what I felt was) a calculated risk. I really thought at that point I knew her well enough to accept his offer.

But I did want (and needed) to pay for some of it, so we shook hands and that was agreed.

Over the next twelve months, the wedding was being organized, and I was still sure I was definitely doing the right thing, or more to the point, I had got the right girl this time from what seemed a decent family. I was going to say 'normal' family, but then what is normal? That's something else I learnt – that average exists but normal is just an interpretation.

So came the wedding day, and at the church I begged my father to behave himself and asked his brother if he wouldn't mind keeping a close eye on him. Unfortunately, my father didn't keep his word, so most of the evening I had one eye on him as he got more and more drunk, and his brother was nearly as bad. Luckily, they had ordered a taxi to take them back home as they were not staying in the same hotel as us. But for the rest of us, the party could carry on, and carry on it did. At last, I could relax knowing that my father wasn't there. In fact, it carried on to nearly 4am in the morning, and finally everyone had worn themselves out and all crawled to bed.

Now this is where things start to get interesting (*or just strange, to me at least*). You see, as I was teetotal then and my new wife wasn't a big drinker either, neither of us was at the point of just passing out on the bed. I can remember my new wife saying that she wanted to open some of the gifts that had been placed in our room and me saying, "No, you must be joking, let's leave them until tomorrow and go to bed. Even though we were both just as tired, I was looking forward to finally being close as we had spent all the time from the church talking to people (new relatives).I know what some of you will be thinking right now (oh yes, he wanted to get his way-that was put politely, wasn't it?) I won't lie – I was looking forward to having intimate relations with my new wife, but we were both so tired and she desperately wanted to sleep (if we were not going to be opening presents,) Which, I must admit, was a bit disappointing and strange if I'm totally being honest, but heyho, we had the rest of our lives to get intimate, so we just slept.

The next day, we were waved off on our way to Cornwall for our honeymoon. But this was disturbing – we only got about 50 miles away from the hotel when we had our first row. By now we had been together just over two years, and until this day, the first day of the honeymoon, we had never had a row. Now, what does that tell you?

Just before the row was sort of over, I said, "Right, we are going back and I'm going to get this marriage annulled." As she looked at me and could see I was serious, I said, "Well, it hasn't been consummated so it can be annulled … ended … that's it. Is that what you want?" Elizabeth then calmed down and said she was sorry and it was just because she was still tired from the last two days. Like a fool, I accepted this. Well, of course I did – I didn't want to believe that I had got it so badly wrong, not again.

Well, we never got to Cornwall. In fact, we only got as far as Poole in Dorset, where we stayed with a relative for a couple of days before going to Elizabeth's family in London for the rest of the week. That was what started the argument, with her wanting to just go to London to see her relatives, not Cornwall, and this would be a cause of arguments in the future. I really couldn't see the fascination with London, and I had worked all over it, but she seemed to have an obsession with the place, and every opportunity she could get to go there, she would. I wouldn't have minded, but she was only one year old when she moved with her parents to Norfolk, so she was hardly hankering after memories.

For the next few months, things were quite difficult, and I don't just mean with Elizabeth and me. I still had a very sporadic work life, and she had lost her job. At that time, we only had my van as transport so she needed to get work either in the village or with transport. After a few months, she finally did get a job at the local hotel, so at least there was some more money coming in, but during this time, I was getting more and more disgruntled with the construction trade, in and out of work all the time. I still wanted to build up a business into a company. I wanted to stand in the front office and look at a fleet of vans and look back and say I built that, but I couldn't see that happening in the building trade. So I decided to go into making plywood linings for the rear inside of vans, as I had done on a number of occasions for my own use. When I looked into this, thinking (rather naively, I admit), *It's a new idea, this is going to be the one*, I found that, although there were many businesses doing just that job, Norfolk and Suffolk seemed to be unrepresented. I could see me being able to grow this business, so I set it up. The only trouble was time is money, and I was running out of both, because I was trying to do everything.

During this time of trying all I could to build this business, we had rented out the bungalow to a tenant and moved in with my in-laws. Now, this actually worked because I would leave to go to my workshop (an old stable) very early when they were all still in bed and wouldn't get home until late, and they would again all be tucked up in bed. So really it wasn't too bad, and it was just to give the business a chance to grow without me needing to draw wages out to pay a mortgage.

But it wasn't enough. I had been working twenty-hour days for over a year now, and it wasn't growing at all – it just seemed to go round in circles. My accountant said I needed a salesperson – someone out there all the time while I concentrated on the rest of the business. He estimated I could get one up and running for around £15,000 – quite a bit of money back in 1996. The only way I could secure this would be by putting my house up for collateral. I did think about it, but not for long. I had fought for the last four years to pay the mortgage to keep the house, just for someone to come and work for me, and then I might still lose the business and I'd also lose the house? No, definitely not.

So I carried on working twenty hours a day doing sales, all the bookwork, cutting, and producing and fitting. I was knackered, but I just kept pushing, trying desperately to get more work and contracts. Suddenly, I couldn't get any money from the bank, and they wouldn't increase the overdraft any further without some form of security. So with a heavy heart, I closed the business and I was gutted. No, I was more than gutted – I was destroyed. I can remember removing the sign-writing from the van in readiness to sell it, and I was so upset, it was like losing a pet. That might sound over the top, but the whole point of writing this book was and is to explore the feelings and thoughts that sometimes are ridiculous but don't seem like it at the time. At the time of whatever is happening, they seem very real. No matter how ridiculous or small to anyone else, they are real.

I had worked my fingers to the bone, and for what? Nothing. I was angry and upset. To me, it wasn't fair – what else could I do? Before too long, especially when the van went, my thoughts were getting the better of me, and to be honest, looking back, I think because I had been working such long hours and trying so hard, my head by then had run out of steam. I could not get things back on track, and I now hadn't any work because I had been out of the jobs market for the last couple of years. I just felt like I was driving into a tunnel – a tunnel without lights, just darkness.

***

I really struggled with what had happened, and my marriage wasn't much better as we seemed to keep arguing. It was like I'd met one person and fallen in love, but once we were married, she'd become a totally different person. I told her this on a number of occasions, and when I did, for a while, I saw that person I'd fallen in love with. It seemed to make sense, but then she would disappear like a ghost until we rowed again, when she would return.

After a few weeks of just sitting in the bedroom and not talking to anyone, after a load of nagging, I finally went to see my doctor, who prescribed me some antidepressants. I took them, but they just didn't make any difference. As I kept driving into the tunnel, it seemed to be getting darker, and I was completely shutting off from everything, just sitting in that room, looking out of the window through the voile curtain and seeing nothing, nothing at all. I returned to the doctors, and he prescribed me some different tablets and also made an appointment for me to see someone from the mental health team. But before that, I started taking the new tablets straight away because the doctor said I could, as they were all anti-depressants and all really in the same family of drugs. Now, I don't know whether he got that wrong as he was only a GP and not a psychiatrist, but when I started these tablets, I can't remember how many I had taken, but it was horrific. I can remember lying on the bed and sweating like I had a fever – sweat was pouring out of me, and I was having the most frightening hallucinations. Not having ever been into drugs, this was a totally new experience to me ,and it was the most scary time I'd ever had. I could see dragons coming at me with fire and snakes with mouths big enough to swallow my head. I couldn't catch my breath, and the more I kept moving, the worse it seem to get.

I kept saying, "Make it stop!" but what could anyone do? While Elizabeth called the doctor, I was flipping around all over the bed like a fish out of water. The hallucinations slowed down, and I managed to lie still, and this seemed to help. The calmer I was, the better they were.

The following day, Elizabeth got an emergency appointment with the on-call psychiatrist, and he prescribed me yet more tablets, saying, "You have just been unlucky with them so far," and with a small grin, he added, "Third time lucky, hey!" To be honest, I couldn't have cared less what he gave me as long as they weren't like the last time. I really just wanted something to knock me out. Don't get me wrong – I wasn't having any problems sleeping. The trouble was upon wakening.

At the time, my father-in-law worked (and we'll use that term loosely) from home and was there 24 hours a day, apart from when he drove my mother-in-law round to the old folks to do home care. But with him at home most of the day and me there, even though I kept in the bedroom, he could not help himself and would keep knocking on the door, saying, "Why don't you come in here with me and we can have a chat over a nice cup of tea?" I'm not sure whether he meant well and had good intentions or if he was lonely, or perhaps it just frustrated him the fact that there was someone in his home who didn't want to talk to him. (In fact, that's not fair to him – at the time, I didn't want to talk to anyone at all, no matter who they were, not even the doctors.) But being him, he would not let it go and kept on and on, asking me or telling me it would do me good to talk, and at the time, I thought, *Yeah, but not to you, now leave me alone.* But that wasn't going to happen, so I said to Elizabeth, "We need to move out – I can't stay here with your dad. We'll have to move back into the bungalow."

So that's what happened, and by the time the tenant had left, the tablets had got a firm hold and I was feeling a little better and a minuscule bit more positive about things.

CHAPTER 14

A harmful mind

Now not having any work I put an ad in the village newsletter and picked up a few small jobs. But I really wasn't keen on getting back into the building trade, so I said, "I think it's time I got out of this for good before we have children. I need to get established in something else."

The only other thing at that time I knew well was training/ fitness. So that was it. But I still had to earn something because my wife's wages didn't cover half of the bills, so I decided to get any old job to tide us over while I got qualified o be a personal trainer/instructor.

I tried my hand at all sorts of things at this point. I was doing some carpentry work for my sister's boyfriend and spoke to a scaffolder on the site, who gave me a job, until he stopped paying me, which I took him to court for. Then I left and got a job in a factory, working as a carpenter on static caravans, which I hated. To me it was like signing into prison on a daily basis, with a tall fence all the way round the perimeter of the site and being searched on your way out every night by the man on the gate. But it was paying money – not much, but more than I had been getting.

Whilst working here and looking into the fitness industry at the local library (no internet in those days), and looking at the pay in that industry, I decided I would try to earn a living at woodcarving. But first, I wanted to get out of the bungalow in the village. If I had sold it, then I would still have owed £5,000 after six years of ownership. So the only answer was to put an extension on it and make it a two-bedroom home – that would get the price up.

So that's what I did. I put an extension right across the back and did as much of the work as I could. I asked my father (when sober) if he could give me a hand with the roof as I physically couldn't pull the trusses up on the walls on my own, and after a bit of groaning, he agreed to help. But that was the only time he ever did anything on any of my houses for me. In fact, he never did anything for me at all as an adult and not too much as a child.

With the extension nearing the end, my father said to me, "Why don't we do some carving together and go to the high-end craft shows?" He had the contacts for carving and was earning a small amount of money from it, when he could be bothered. But more often than not, I would end up finishing one of his jobs after working all day. So I said I would think about it. After a while, I said, "As long as you put in as much as me, then yes, let's do it."

By this time, my father's drinking was under some sort of control. By 'control', I mean instead of going two or three days without any drink at all and being intolerable, groaning around like a bear with a sore head, snapping and shouting all the time, he was now drinking every evening continually, seven days a week. This meant no benders and no massively aggressive behaviour, wanting to kill people. So that was better for family relations, and as long as I'd left before he was on about his sixth can of lager, there would be no trouble for me. I did say, "This is your chance to make things better, please don't screw it up." You see, by now, I'd been working on my own and with other builders and had started to form my own opinions, my own ideas – gradually, I was (pardon the cliché) 'finding myself'. I needed to, because up to the point of getting married, I was still his puppet, doing what I was told and even defending his opinions.

Anyway, we did the carving business, and I sorted the designing part, got the business cards, leaflets, *etc*. I did most of the work, in fact, which was not a surprise. But my father, when not drunk, could talk the hind legs off a donkey, and as I was still far from gregarious and really not comfortable being in front of a crowd, I needed him, and I really wanted to still build up a business. But I should have known better. Not only did I do 90% of the work setting the business up, making a stand to trade from, and carving a sign, I also organized getting everything together for our first show.

For sales, it was a disaster. Come to that, so were the second and third shows (the shows were all over the country). "Well, that's it, then. That didn't work, hey?" my father said. But I said, "No, as far as selling it didn't, but I think we need to go back to the promoters and tell them instead of paying *them* for a stand, they should be paying *us*." You see, with me out front on a bench carving constantly, people were fascinated at watching this, and I must have had twenty to thirty people crowded round me permanently all day whilst my father was answering questions. That was what we need to be doing and getting paid for, but he wasn't interested, and I knew I couldn't do this on my own. So with that and a heavy heart, we returned to Norfolk.

So where was I now? Back to square one – left the job, no other work, no business … I really felt down and at this point thinking that the same answer was in my head again and spending quite some time thinking of the best way I could conduct the self-termination. (Warning, the next paragraph could be triggering) I came up with a sure way involving a noose (I'm not going to detail this plan for the obvious reasons), formed it with a length of rope, and left it behind my seat for what would have been nearly three years or so – always as an answer in case the situation just become non-tenable to me and the anger was strong enough. Unfortunately, down was the way I was heading, just trying to keep afloat. I reluctantly started working on bits and bobs, drifting along, and at this time, I had finally sold the bungalow. My first property that I had extended sold at last for the same price as it had cost me, plus the extension cost, so I made nothing after eight years, all thanks to the housing market crashing and the government at the time. But on the bright side, I was moving, starting afresh, and had decided after a lot of arguing with my wife to buy a brand new house in the next village. If I'm completely honest, I wasn't too sure about it, but it was a lovely house and there not much I had to do with it (I was again looking to get out of building). The trouble was, at the time, I needed to be busy. And even though it was a busy few weeks around the move, once we were in, I still hadn't any work to speak of, and I was slipping again.

***

Elizabeth and I had been married now for around four years, and the year previously I'd talked to her about her coming off the pill. At the time, she replied, "Do you think now is the right time?" My Nanna told me after having five children around the Second World War that there is never a right time – if you wait for the right time, you will miss the boat, as it were.

I said, "We both want children, so let's try. You don't know, it might take two years before we conceive, but just come off the pill and we'll see what happens."

She said she would, and in the meantime, she said she'd like to get a dog. Straight away, I retorted, "Not instead of a baby, I hope," but she assured me it wasn't. According to her, she wanted some company and something to do when I worked away from home.

She said, "It's boring here on my own," and fair enough – the village didn't have a lot going on. (In fact, very soon after we had moved, I quickly realised it was the wrong place to live, at least for me.) So we got a black Labrador puppy, which I named Mad Max, or Max for short. I called him Mad Max because he was so lively. He literally was pinging of the walls – absolutely bonkers. So it was Mad Max or Tigger or Bouncer.

Getting him did lift the mood for a while, but it didn't lift it far. By now we had been in the house for just over six months, and I was back in that tunnel again with nothing around me to look at, just darkness heading into further darkness. I really couldn't see a way out at all. I was by now under the mental health team again, albeit in a different council borough, and had a CPN (Community Psychiatric Nurse) visiting weekly with monthly tablet reviews at the hospital. But even with this, I wasn't getting better, and they weren't listening to me, or that was my perception at the time. When I did say something, they were not hearing me, so I was just spiralling downward.

One day, the nurse had his supervisor with him. Something was said, and they then excused themselves and were talking in my kitchen whilst I was sitting in the lounge. They asked to speak with my wife on her own. Then they all came back into the lounge and sat down looking at me. The supervisor said, "James, we would like to admit you to hospital for your own safety, but under the Mental Health Act, we need you to sign a voluntary section notice for us will you do that?"

I looked across to Elizabeth as she just nodded, and I asked what would happen if I refused. The supervisor said, "We would have to get an order from a psychiatrist to have you sectioned under the Mental Health Act." So I agreed to go to hospital.

When in the hospital, I was lucky enough to have a room instead of being on the ward, but even so, as a nurse led me off to the room, there were faces all looking and staring, making various noises. It felt like more of a zoo environment than a hospital (although there was that hospital smell of antiseptic and Jey's cleaning fluid) – it was how the others in the ward responded to the newcomer, like a new monkey coming into their enclosure. That was just how it felt – very primitive. The patients would all stick together in their groups, and I wonder now as I write this whether that was because of where they were (a natural instinct, as such) or because of their illnesses or something else. I was strangely conflicted because about 10% of me felt self-preservation kicking in, and I was threatened by this environment, despite the psychiatrist trying to reassure me I was in the best place. But really, I couldn't have cared less what they did or didn't do with me. I really was past caring and past hoping, to be completely honest.

Another reason why they felt I needed to be in hospital was because I couldn't look after myself. Just simple tasks seemed so complicated, so I wouldn't bother with them. Not caring to me meant not doing, and when, for example, the nurse said to clean my teeth, I had to really study the toothpaste and brush before then trying to work out what to do with it. But once I got started, I was ok, and it then seemed simple. At this point, I think they were worried that I had suffered some kind of stroke, but after some tests, it turned out that my brain had simply decided to shut down. (This is what they term as a 'mental breakdown', not a 'nervous breakdown', as it's the mind/brain and not the nervous system that leads to it. Or as they put it, "It's your brain's way of having a rest.")

You see, I'm by nature an over-thinker and am constantly thinking of one thing or another and never really shutting off at all. This behaviour, uncontrolled, can lead to a mental breakdown. One thing they were concerned about was to what level I had broken down. I suppose, had I been in a different place mentally and had any understanding or any sense of caring about what was happening, I would have been worried, but as it was, being in a depressive state stopped any concerns or worries. To be frank, I really couldn't have cared less about what had happened at all. In fact, it was a bit of a relief. When I'd slipped into this tunnel before, I was still very conscious of the fact that I was sitting at home looking into darkness, metaphorically speaking, and still aware that I wasn't earning any money at all, nothing. (Self-employed people in the UK were, back then, told to go to the DSS – Department for Social Services, but more often than not, when asking for help, we got: "Tough!" As if we were being persecuted for standing on our own two feet.) It's ironic really because you would have thought they'd support independent people who were/are no burden on the state whatsoever. But no! Not in the UK.

Somehow, even in a severe clinical depression, I was aware of this situation and knew that the longer I was out of action, the more debt was building. I would pay wages from my business account to the mortgage account (a joint account at the time). So at least the mortgage was never in arrears. But my business account obviously would be, and when and if I got back, I would have to work like a Trojan to pay it off. I hasten to add that I always did work hard, as a point of principle. With this burden in my forward conscience it was incredibly frustrating, like having a mind split in two, because I knew I needed to be working, but the depression didn't give a hoot about that and wouldn't budge. So the only hope was that the tablets could raise the levels of serotonin in my brain to get me to the edge of the depression so at least I could function again. As many of you out there will know, depression is selfish and it really couldn't care less about your financial situation. But in itself, the financial situation it puts you in makes the depression worse again – it's a vicious circle, and still the depression doesn't care! Or does it? One for later on.

But this time, in hospital, I had plenty of cares to worry about, but I didn't. I wasn't worried about the money … wasn't worried about my wife or our new addition, Max … I just couldn't think of anything – it was like being a zombie. I could see things around me, I could see other residents playing pool on the pool table in the recreation area but couldn't play myself. It was surreal, like I was a ghost and could see but not touch, or at least, I just couldn't get my brain or mind to think on what to do next and send a message to my body.

This was how it was for just over a week or so, and then for no apparent reason, things changed. I woke one morning to some commotion going on in the ward, where security had been called, and as I peeked through the door, I saw it was one of the patients having a schizophrenic episode. I could hear noises and sounds that I previously hadn't heard (or rather hadn't registered), and now I could hear where I was, and for the first time in what had seemed like months, but actually was only around seven days, I had a thought, and not just a negative, unhelpful thought but a constructive thought. And that thought was: *I shouldn't be here.* You see, I was put on a ward with patients who all had disorders of the mind like schizophrenia, but at the time, I was being treated for depression, not a disorder.

I really think doctors should re-name mental disorders with the term 'disorder of the mind'. In fact, I think from my experiences, they should try to replace the term 'mental' with something that doesn't conjure up images and thoughts of 'nutters' or 'nut-houses' – an old term that I still hear today. This does nothing for the people like me who suffer on a daily basis, in varying degrees, with illnesses of the mind. But hey, that's my opinion.

Getting back again to the room I was in – it had buttons instead of pull cords for lighting and no grab rails anywhere, and even the mirror wasn't glass, yet the door and window were (strange I had that thought as I was leaving the room, hopefully for good). As I left the ward, I still had this sort of haze around in my head and the feeling of detachment was still evident, but I knew I didn't want to be there any longer. I wanted out of there, but I also wanted out from the outside world. In other words, I did still have thoughts and plans for self-termination.

The doctors were deeply concerned that, once out of their care, I may do something and were very reluctant to let me leave, only doing so on an absolute agreement that I would attend the hospital on a daily basis until they felt I was safe to be left alone. In a strange way, I understood, because at the point of being put into hospital with what was diagnosed as a mental breakdown, I actually would have been just as safe at home. This is because the thoughts of suicide just weren't there at that time. Quite simply, I had no thoughts ... of anything. It was *now*, when the thought process was appearing to get back on track, that I could harm myself, simply because I *was* thinking.

Elizabeth picked me up and we went home. Thoughts of money were now coming into my head, and the debts were building again. To add to this, Elizabeth had to take time off to drive me to the hospital every day, so she wasn't working either. If anything was going to knock you over the edge, it would be this.

For a number of weeks, I visited the hospital on a daily basis and talked to the psychiatrist, a psychologist, and number of psychiatric nurses, and my mood was starting to lift. After talking to one of the nurses one day, I decided that work was a big problem in my life (as it is in everyone's life, but for different reasons) and I should do more of the work I liked doing, instead of just chasing the pound.

CHAPTER 15

Working too hard, but still standing!

One of the things I liked doing was driving, so what about driving people around? Long story short, I looked into this, and it seemed like a good idea. The pros that I could see at the time outweighed the cons, and off I went and started a taxi business.

Setting this up kept me busy and motivated, and before long I was trading. Now there was one factor that I definitely didn't see coming, or anyone else come to that, but I don't know why we all missed it – and that was that a lot of the fares were from pubs. If it was women, there were no problems, but drunken males … If you remember, I didn't deal with drunken men at all well – it angered me to such an extent that, for their safety (and me not ending up in prison), I would have to leave immediately… but this isn't possible when they are in your car.

However, by now, thanks to my father-in-law, I had learned that not all males responded to alcohol in the same way. Some in fact could be quite entertaining (well, entertaining to me). But my biggest difficulty was with was the aggressive ones. I really could not (and if I'm completely honest, didn't want to) get my head round these idiots, as I see them.

For a number of other reasons, I decided to close the taxi business after only a few weeks, for the sake of my mind's health *(that's what I'll call it rather than 'mental health')*. I was still taking the medication, and that seemed to be keeping me buoyant. So

I quickly moved on and swapped the taxi car for a van and returned to the building trade once again.

***

Whilst all this was going on, we (my wife and I) had moved again and made a little money this time. The house I bought had a big enough garden for me to double the size of the property, but after drawing all the plans and finally getting permission, she told me she didn't want me to do all that work. Why couldn't we just buy a house the right size that just needed painting, even if we had to increase the mortgage? (I might add, I had just reduced the mortgage, much to her disgust.) I just couldn't get it through to her that borrowing is fine if, and *only* if, you have the ability to pay it back. She never did grasp that, and that was probably why I was constantly robbing my business account to bail out our private account that she ran. So in the end, after continual arguing day after day, I agreed I would extend to try to make a profit, and we again would move. But in the end, the extension didn't happen. We had to stay for a while because of serious health problems with our dog, Max. At only 12 weeks old, I took him to the vets for a routine injection, and the head vet diagnosed him with severe dysplasia in both rear hips. I remember the vet asking me what I wanted to do, and I was a bit bemused by the question. He told me I wouldn't get any insurance for the dog now that he had made this diagnosis. He asked, "Do you want to leave him with me?"

I knew what he meant. And I said "No … I don't, I made a commitment to this dog, took him away from his siblings, and I'm not going to abandon him now, no matter what." So I had to build a run for Max and a pen in the house, and he needed to finish his treatments before we moved again. Yet again, this didn't go down well with Elizabeth, but that was how it was ,and this time I was going to stick to my guns.

It was around this time that I met someone I used to know as a child and ended up getting a £250k contract from him. I felt this was the time I could finally build a company. With all this work, I was employing different people, and even though it was the building trade again, I was finally creating a business – with two vans. It was a start. The downfall was the fact that, to keep these men in work and keep other jobs running, I was working twenty-hour days again, and this was having a detrimental effect on my health, both my body and my mind. I was constantly running from job to job, more often than not putting things right, to my standard. I was running myself into the ground and I couldn't see it. In fact, on the contrary – I thought I was buzzing.

One morning, I got to a bungalow that was empty, and we were re-fitting for a lady. I hadn't even been to bed that night and turned up at 6 am to get a few things done before the men got there when I heard a knock. As I went to the door and looked out up the drive to see the owner arriving I suddenly turned and collapsed on the front step in front of her Fortunately, the lady in question was a nurse and knew exactly what to do. After spending a number of hours in the local hospital, I was finally released and told to calm things down.

Calm things down? How was I supposed to do that? This was me, I thought – or was it? I did have the next day off. Due to a dispute with the main contractor, I'd quit that work anyway (strict principles again) and lost four out of the five men I had full time. I decided, *Enough is enough – I'm out, no matter what.* So I sold all my equipment. I guess I was trying to burn my bridges to make sure I couldn't go back. I think I needed to do that at that time. I just kept enough tools for home projects and booked myself on a YMCA training course to become a gym instructor/personal trainer.

I wound down the building works and started training seriously, getting myself back into shape – not that I was out of shape, but I just needed to feel in the right place. For the next few weeks, I got a job in a gym (no payment, unfortunately – just for the experience). Then I went to London, stayed with a member of my wife's family, and got myself qualified as an instructor/personal trainer. By the time this had happened, we were on the move to a new house, which was big enough for us two, Max, and any additions that might turn up. (On this point, I was starting to get concerned that we may have a problem, but at present, I was too busy with all these other events.)

After a short while, I got a job in a gym, but it was only part-time and they were going to take too long for it to become full-time. So I got another job that was full-time but on shifts. This didn't bother me at all as most of the time my wife and I were together was spent arguing anyway, so it was quite nice coming home when she was going to work and I could be with Max. Because we still hadn't had a child, I was very close to Max indeed and very protective. He basically was my child, just in a furry coat and never likely to grow up – he was full of it, bouncing around. But could behave if food was in the equation.

Working in the gym didn't really help our relationship because Elizabeth was really jealous of female clients and colleagues. Whenever I came back from a shift, she'd ask who I had been talking to – "Bet they were pretty, bet they were slim," – and on and on – she would not let this go. I did say one thing to her in response, and that was, "At least they listen to me, unlike you!" As you can imagine, this went down like a lead balloon.

When I worked as a boy on building sites, the older men, all different trades, often tried to give advice, for example: "Don't p**s all your wages up the wall" (well, that one wasn't going to affect me since I didn't drink) and "Put your money in bricks and mortar" (that one didn't turn out so well, as I lost £20,000 in less than six months – thanks for that advice. Good job I can't remember who gave me that little nugget.) But there was also this one, which I did listen to: "If you want to see what your future wife will look like in twenty years time, look at her mother." So when I got to meet the future mother-in-law and thought, *Wow, she is nice*, I also thought, *If Elizabeth looks like that in twenty years time, I will be more than happy*. Not that looks mean anything, and at the time, I think I was referring more to her mother's behaviour than looks. Thinking she was going to be the same in her behaviour, but sadly (for me) she was a carbon copy of her father in her behaviours and attitudes.

Unfortunately, my wife may have inherited her mother's good-looking genes, but she was argumentative in the extreme, just like her father. She would not listen and thought she knew all the answers, at least when it suited her. The good points about him (the father in-law) were he had a great sense of humour and we had some good laughs together. Sadly, Elizabeth did not have that skill at all and rarely, if ever, made me laugh. It was usually me making her laugh. That's ironic from a man constantly being diagnosed with depression, hey! Another way she was like her father was never wanting to go anywhere – well, apart from shopping. That included not wanting to go abroad on holiday (she wouldn't fly and wouldn't go on a boat – she never told me *that* before we got married …).

Anyway, after over three and a half months of earache from her while I worked at the gym, I had a phone call from an old trade friend who offered me about two months' work. When he said the rate (which happened to be about double what I was getting in the gym), I said, "Yes, when do you need me to start?" The manager of the gym let me go without working any notice, and I said I would start the new job the next Monday. And that was that.

So when I got home and Elizabeth asked as usual who I had talked to, I said, "Just stop there – you haven't got to worry about who I talk to in the gym any longer because I've just quit the job!" I thought she would be pleased, but no. She just said, "Well, that was clever – what are we going to do for money now?" And before I could say anything, it was followed with, "I suppose it's on me again." Which was ironic because it was *my* business account that was *always* bailing her out of debt.

Well, to say I was steaming would be putting it mildly. But under control, I simply walked away, with her and her arguments following me. I could have told her about the other job, and had the response been different I would have, but I thought, *You don't deserve that information, not until Sunday or Monday, depending how the weekend goes.*

So I was back in the building trade again after the house move – this time, we were in a bigger town and living on what was meant to be one of the better developments. I worked for the friend I mentioned earlier for a number of weeks, and then the customer asked me if I would stay on, work directly for him, and refurbish the remainder of the cottage he lived in. I hadn't any other work, and my friend was ok about it, so I agreed. I was there mostly on my own, and day after day of this was starting to get to me. Too much time on my own wasn't good for an over-thinker – it was very easy for the negative thoughts to take over, and that was really bad for me. But I needed to earn a living.

So I carried on until I'd finished the project, but unfortunately for the customer, a dear man with a lovely manner, he had been diagnosed with Motor Neurone Disease and was basically dying in front of me. It wasn't long before he passed on. This had a profound effect on me since it was only a year and a half since I'd lost another customer – another dear man who only wanted to do right. Once, I was sitting in his sitting room after I'd made him a cup of tea when he said, "If you want to do something, don't leave it, James – just do it." And within a week of him saying this, he had died.

But the customer who I lost and had the most profound effect on me was a surgeon and his wife, who was a nurse. He was ill when I first worked for them and got worse. After a dreadful time coping with her husband, she herself was diagnosed with terminal cancer.

This really played with my head. How could life be so unfair? These people hadn't hurt anyone, and in fact I thought often, *How many lives has that surgeon saved, and his nurse wife? And that's the payback – both dead before they were seventy.* These sorts of happenings would make me question many things, and not being able to get answers that made sense, I really struggled with the rights and wrongs of life.

Anyway, we were living in the new house, and during this time, my father decided he wanted to split from my mother after thirty-four years. He decided he was going to make a new life in France – I thought, *France, why France?* because he had always said he hated the French. He told me as a child that they and the Italians were a bunch of cowards and he always favoured the Germans. So why France? Well, I would say because they are a drinking nation, but not like the Brits who are known for being a bunch of binge drinkers. The French way of life seems to be more conducive to somebody with a liking for heavy drinking, so what better place to be, hey? (In France, he could hide is addiction very easily.)

So they split and he went off to France. My mother, however, returned to the town of Bury St. Edmunds, where she had grown up and where *her* family lived (a mother and two sisters at the time). But probably just over a year later, my father suddenly turned up on my doorstep with this huge old worn-out camper van and announced that he had returned. By now, I'd had enough time away from him that he hadn't any influence on me at all. Although I was still trying to establish who I was, I was definitely more assured in front of him and wasn't about to go back to having him bully me. I invited him in (as it's the polite thing to do) and then said, "So, what are you doing here?" He just said things weren't working in France and he thought he might have made a mistake. So I said, "Right, you can stay here, but you do not under any circumstances come back to *my* house drunk, and remember, this is *my* house not yours, so you live here under *my* rules."

For the first two weeks, we were all dodging along, but I did have to remind him a couple of times, even in those two weeks, whose home he was staying in. But then, wham! He came back one night, or rather early morning (when he said he was just visiting his mother), as drunk as could be – absolutely paralytic, lumping and banging around. It had been many years that since I'd lived with him and a few years since I'd seen him in this state. But as I stood on my landing and contemplated going down to physically throw him out of my home (which was something I really wanted to do), the heart started racing and the memories of my youth began washing round my head. I could feel my chest tightening and my breathing starting to labour as I turned and went back into the bedroom (I did, however, call my boy Max upstairs and put him in the bedroom for safe keeping). I sat on the end of the bed with my head in my hands and was so annoyed with myself. This was my house, not his, and I was a fully-grown man, nearly six inches taller than him and probably ten inches wider at the shoulders, but I couldn't confront him. I hate to admit it, but it was like I'd gone back to being that boy, and I was still scared – but just of him. Not of other drunken males that, over my late teens/early twenties, I'd had a few 'skirmishes' with – it was just him. As I sat there, I said to Elizabeth, "This is ridiculous." I was so angry with myself, but that was it, and he eventually quietened and went to bed.

In the morning, I went to work, but I was still not happy with working back where I had desperately been trying to get away from. I thought I liked the driving part of the taxi business, but it was the people part that was the problem, so what about taking my HGV license? This seemed like a good idea. In fact, it seemed like the idea I'd been waiting for. I would be away from home all week, so no arguments with Elizabeth and only seeing each other at weekends – that should surely help with the relationship. The thought of driving something so big didn't faze me at all; after all, driving was something I was (and still am) 100% confident in, no matter the circumstances.

I was still seeing a CPN once a week at the local clinic and having something called Cognitive Behavioural Therapy (CBT with a psychologist). (That was, when the nurse could concentrate on the job and stop asking me questions about DIY for his own home projects). I ran the HGV idea by the CPN, and on the surface, he thought it to be a good idea too. So I got an application form, went to my doctor for the medical, and sent it off, waiting in anticipation. Nearly a month later, I got a letter from the DVLA, but instead of it being my provisional licence for the HGV training to start, it was a notice of the cessation of my entitlement to drive. I had been banned from driving altogether from midnight previous because of the amount and type of anti-depressants I was taking. (In fact, they were not the regular anti-depressant, they were a new type called SSRIs (Selective Serotonin Re-Uptake Inhibitors). These where helping me keep things rational; they were like a calming effect instead of getting so desperately frustrated, to give you time to think – ironic, really!

I could not believe this. I knew I suffered from bad luck (or rather, my perception was that I was very unlucky as a person, and this thought is *very* relevant), but this was ridiculous. Now I could not drive anywhere, and if I did and was stopped, the ban could be extended. I was in the middle of a kitchen refurbishment as well, and now I couldn't get anywhere, and all because I was taking a type of antidepressant to try and help myself get better – well, thanks very much. The ban was for four months, initially. But a letter from the psychiatrist confirmed that I would be fine to drive cars. But I still wasn't allowed to drive an HGV, so that idea was out of the window because I really couldn't see myself getting off the tablets any time soon.

Going back to my father, who had twice now come back to my house drunk. Unlike when I was young, I sat him down and told him it couldn't happen again (not that saying anything to him would change anything, because he was the type who only heard what he wanted to, so really I was wasting my breath). But the third time he came back paralytically drunk, the following afternoon (as he was in bed all the morning) .I said, "Right, I want you to leave by the end of the week."

I started to see a psychologist on a regular basis for CBT, instead of the CPN, who wasn't really focussed enough to do me any good. By then, I think the penny had dropped with the mental health team that it wasn't depression *per se* that needed addressing – it was my thinking and mindset, which was something I had been saying for a number of years. I was sure it was my thoughts and feelings that triggered the depression, and *not* the other way round. Up till then, they just kept treating me for depression, and then when my mood was more buoyant, they would sign me off.

But here I was for the umpteenth time, still suffering, and it wasn't getting any easier. I had so many thoughts and feelings and perceptions that my head was spinning nearly all day, and if it wasn't for the tablets, I wouldn't have been sleeping at all. It was only when I was in a deep depression that I really slept well. I suppose it was like living your life riding a roller-coaster – full of ups and downs. But it wasn't like being bi-polar (still called manic depression back then). My sister was like that – one day, she was pinging off the walls and the next she would be very down (not depressed, just down in the dumps). When she was pinging, it was unbearable. I was never anything like that. Mine was deeper – much deeper than what I had seen of my sister's behaviour.

One of the things we discussed was a deeply held belief about 'correct' behaviour. All the way through my childhood, I was told in no uncertain terms that swearing was completely forbidden, in the house, garden, and at work. My father actually told me that "swearing was for people who didn't have the intelligence to find an alternative to the swear word." This pressure to never swear at all when all my peers did (and, in fact, so did nearly everyone I ever come across) was quite immense. But as I was told by him that it was not acceptable at all, that was how it had to be.

***

I didn't swear until I first started seeing this psychologist, who I knew was far more educated and intelligent than my father. She explained to me that it was fine to swear if it was needed and that she would often swear at her boyfriend. But you see how the brainwashing and bullying can take such a hold if it is started young? I did find it immensely hard at first to swear without feeling guilty for what I had just said. It was just another part of the emotional conditioning that was not helping in my life.

The despair I felt had led me to a new discovery. You see, the things I have written about (the things going wrong, or my perception that things kept going wrong) are only the tip of the iceberg. Even others would say to me (and this really didn't help at all): "You don't have much luck, do you?"

At this time, I now had my licence back, and the van that I had just bought from a reputable dealer was playing up seriously. I was working with an uncle of mine who always had time for me now that I was an adult. For some reason, the situation was making me feel very despondent. One day, when we were having lunch and had been talking about the van problems, I made a flippant remark to my uncle. I found myself saying, "I don't know what I've done in a past life, but it must have been bad to deserve this – I reckon I must have raped a whole village!"

Silence fell around us as we just sat there looking out of the windscreen to the fields, and then my uncle said, "I'll bring you a book tomorrow that will explain everything." I asked him what he meant and he said, "Do you believe in reincarnation? Do you really believe you are being punished for something you did, or rather something your last being did?"

First, I thought, *Woo, is this a religious belief? What is he talking about?* He said to me, "I'll bring you the book. You read it. I think it'll help you understand more about how things work."

So the next day, he did. We were nearly finished on this job, but I needed to read this book, so I stayed at home for the last day and read it from cover to cover. Wow – how interesting and disturbing at the same time! But unfortunately, the disturbing part was now running at full speed round my head. You see, it did indeed say that we are all reincarnated from a past life, and, according to the book and the spiritualist church, if a past being has been bad, then the next one reincarnated has to make amends. But when the incarnated one has died and lived their life of nothing but good, their next being will have a good life, unless they decide to go the bad way. There were short but detailed stories of people who had been reincarnated and knew each other when they first met without uttering a single word – romances between people who knew things about another that nobody could have known. This book worryingly made so much sense to me, but *How unfair!* I thought. *Why should I have to pay back for someone else's misdemeanours?*

By now, the romanticism of the long-lost couple was diminishing rapidly, and this payback issue was now dominating my mind. In fact, I could barely think of anything else at all. I just kept thinking how unfair it was, wondering how can I stop this? I worried I was going to be paying this debt until the day I died so the next human being reincarnated from me could have a good life. But what about *my* life?

This situation really started to anger me deeply, and I decided to speak to the psychologist that I was seeing on a fortnightly basis, but she didn't believe in reincarnation. It had only been a couple of weeks before when we were talking about 'the grey areas' – I was just seeing everything, every situation, in black or white without any allowance for grey at all, which was another belief/behaviour that I had to address. Yet when I mentioned reincarnation, she firmly said, "There is no such thing! How can there be? If there was such a thing as reincarnation, the amount of people on the planet would stay the same." Her opinion about that was very black and white and actually completely wrong, as it would depend on how many children the incarnated actually had, which would/could change the population.

At the time, I never argued or said any more about this to

her. But once on my own, I was thinking about nothing else. Reincarnation could be true – it made sense, but I was dammed if I was going to pay back a debt to fate for something I hadn't done. The trouble was, how could I stop this persecution? Well, there was only one answer. Nothing at that time was good, apart from my dog. Work, the trouble with my father, my marriage … (which, really, I knew I needed to end but just didn't have the strength or conviction to.) And something else – when I was ill, Elizabeth seemed to be much happier. I put this down to the fact that she could do whatever she liked without any questioning, even getting us into debt because I wasn't really around, not mentally, anyway. What a life – it just seemed an endless round of misery.

So I had my new information, and I was now convincing myself that *really* everyone would be better off without me and I would definitely be better off without the world. And the same answer kept coming up every time, and that was self-termination. I would look around me at the way people treated each other, and in my opinion, it was getting a whole lot worse than the previous twenty /thirty years. You know, back when everyone had time to say good morning to everyone else and children had respect for the police (probably driven by fear, but still). People on the whole were more respectful of each other. To me, it was a better time all round, and I often wished I had been born during the forties to experience the fifties and sixties first-hand. I really struggled with this greedy and selfish world. I really didn't want to be part of what was present or what was coming, so in my head, I was sure that self-termination was the only way of finally stopping the pain. You see, if things in your life bring you pain, you can move away from them, and to a degree, if the body gives you pain, you can repair it with a bandage or similar, but if the mind is giving you pain, there isn't any escape from it, apart from taking drugs or getting blind drunk. There just isn't any place to go, and I was too much of a pragmatic person to think that a quick high was going to solve anything. But what I had decided was that I would have the last say. I would finally be in control of my life. It was just a shame it was right at the end of it, but still, I would be in control at last.

CHAPTER 16

And the worst was to come

On a late spring morning, after my wife had gone to work and I had told her that I had a migraine (which I've always suffered with since I was nine years old), I got up and walked my dog, Max, in the forest that now I was planning to be my last place of living. As I was looking for a suitable place, he was running about, totally oblivious to what his Dad was planning. I got him back into the car and drove him home, where I sat at my desk and wrote a letter for Elizabeth to see once the deed was done and then left the letter on the kitchen table. I looked back at my boy, and the tears just streamed down my face as I hugged him and told him how sorry I was, but it was something I had to do. I gave him his favourite chew, which was a Jumbone.

I then went to the garage, got a pile of rags, and the garden hose pipe and put them in the car, then set off to the place I had earmarked earlier.

I parked up close to the bushes and remember getting out and placing the hose up the exhaust pipe and then stuffing some of the rag up around the hose. Then I pulled the hose round from the back of the car to the front window, and I opened it just enough to put the hose through. Then using the rags again, I stuffed the rest of the opening of the window and got back in the car, in the driver's seat (out of habit). I turned the engine on and gave the accelerator a push, just to make sure the hose or rags weren't going to fall out.

I just sat there, and within seconds, I was sobbing, thinking about my dog and the fact that I'd left him – I loved him like a child. I can remember I kept saying, "Sorry, mate, I'm really sorry." Then within a few minutes, there was an iron-like taste, and I had just started feeling a bit light-headed and then a little sick.

Suddenly, out of nowhere, a van pulled up about 50 feet away, and as I looked in my mirror, feeling even more sick and light-headed, his door opened and he then moved toward my car. With that, I put my foot straight to the floor and tore through the hedge across the grass and headed for the main road, down the forest track. It wasn't till I got to a clearing just before the main road that I stopped, but I didn't wait around – I got out of the car and pulled the hose and rags from the window, stuffed them into the boot, then drove away. At this point, and not really in a fit state to drive, I felt rather ill, so had to pull over to be sick.

Once back in the car, I just sat there, looking out of the screen but feeling totally detached from what was around me, and the emotions were almost overwhelming. I was angry I chose that spot ... but it was right off the main forest track about a mile and a half in the forest – how would anyone know there was a car there? And then out of nowhere, a van turned up. Why did he come that far into the forest? It just didn't make sense ... well, not initially. But after a while, it became clear to what levels fate was determined to preserve me and continue the persecution.

After about 20 minutes, I started the car and slowly drove back to my house, where I picked up my dog and headed straight back out to another end of the forest, just to walk and think about what had just happened and what to do next. As my boy sniffed his way along the forest track and I watched him, I knew that, as much as I loved him, it wasn't enough. I felt he was the only thing I had worth living for, but it *still* wasn't enough. I felt very frustrated and trapped, and one of the saddest parts was that the forest that, as a child, had held me and comforted me so much was now being associated with misery, frustration, and anger. I felt I had nowhere to go. We walked for the best part of two hours before returning to the car, but I still didn't want to be at home, so I just drove around, parking up here and there, and looking at the world go by, feeling totally numb.

Then my phone rang , and it was Elizabeth asking about the letter she had found on the kitchen table. I totally forgot about that when I picked Max up, and now she knew what I'd planned to do. She told me to come straight home – she had got an emergency appointment with the mental health team. So I returned and we went straight to the hospital.

Now the problem was that I was already on the maximum dosage I could have of an anti-depressant that worked for me, and the only way from here drug-wise was going to be Valium. I'd heard it had quite a few side effects that weren't pleasant, and I really didn't think there would be any benefit of taking this drug. As I'd said to them, it was the thoughts and misery that drove the anger to want to get out of life.

I said, "I am not depressed – I am angry, and that anger is the driving force." They said that the Venlafaxine should temper that anger and make me feel calmer, and I told them it did, but clearly not enough. Which led them back to Valium. I agreed in the end to trial it for a while and see how I felt.

But Valium sent me completely the other way and turned me into a zombie, unable to do anything apart from feed myself and go to the toilet. So I stopped taking it, which was quite a relief, and in a strange sort of way I felt a bit better in myself.

But when talking to the psychologist, she would say, "How do you feel?" Being in the depths of despair, I would think, *What a stupid question.* My facial expressions have always given away my inner thoughts – it's a bugger trying to lie when you have an honest face, always a giveaway

I once said to her that I felt like I was flying a plane on my own (just a small one) and was desperately trying to get above the trees of the forest below, but then it would start to nose dive and I would have an incredible struggle to stop it from crashing into the mountain ahead. I suppose being on the Venlafaxine helped my ability to handle the plane, in the sense of keeping it in the sky, albeit very close to the obstacles that kept getting in the way.

***

We were moving again, but this time it was because my garage and van had been broken into and all my tools and equipment were stolen. We hadn't had too much trouble where we were, but this was the final straw, so ironically, I found a house for sale in the village where we had started our marriage. Yes, I know they say you shouldn't go back, but it seemed like the right thing to do. It was a three-bed detached that was in need of 'refurbishment', but it turned out to be more of a complete renovation.

As we packed to move and a date was set, I was out walking Max one day when I got back home to hear someone talking on the phone in the spare room, which was my office. As I looked up the stairs, my wife poked her head round the door frame and whispered, "It's your dad."

"Oh, right," I said and picked up the other phone in the hallway downstairs, where I could listen or join in. And what I heard was my father actually slagging me off to Elizabeth, saying all I needed was a "kick up the arse" and I should get off those tablets. Obviously, he was drunk – no change there, then. So I told him to get off my phone and never call us again, ever. I really hit the roof, especially when Elizabeth tried to defend him. "NO!" I said, "Enough is enough, and he has crossed the line for the last time."

For a while, he did call a number of times, and if I was at home, I would just hang up on him after telling him not to call me again. For the first couple of Christmases, he sent a card, but if I got to it first, I would not even open it. I'd just burn it. Then it all stopped and no further contact was had.

So we moved house, and I quickly got to work planning and drawing out how to alter the house for the best. By then, I was working in the building trade again but was feeling a little more positive about things as I could see this house finally funding a building plot outright and, at last, a mortgage free life, but first things first was to get the house sorted. At this point, I was still taking the maximum dosage of the antidepressants or SSRIs. To note, SSRIs are a different form of antidepressant but listed as antidepressants in the UK (later on, I explain what the letters stand for). and trying desperately to concentrate on other things. And so I was now working round the clock, and being busy was good (sort of).

My marriage was still very fractious and really not too good, but it never had been, and after 10 years, we were still childless, which was something else that affected my mood. I thought, *Why is this not happening?* I suppose, having sex only twice a year was somewhat impeding the chances. The trouble was that when the subject came up, it always caused arguments and tears, but things always did improve once all had been said – well, for a short while, before reverting back to the status quo.

I decided that it was time to take action on the matter as Elizabeth seemed quite happy just to plod along, even though she would insist that she did still want children and was as concerned as I was. Well, I thought she had a funny way of showing it. And because I'm proactive person and do not really believe in just waiting for something to happen, I booked an appointment with our GP. He agreed for me to take a fertility test, which I did, and found there was nothing wrong with me. I then had to persuade Elizabeth to have tests too, but I said, "We are both in our 30s and childless. You said you wanted four children – we are running out of time."

So she agreed to go to the GP and take the tests, but I wasn't with her, so I had to take her word for it when she said they were normal too. So I said, "So it must be that we have to up our game, yes?" She agreed verbally, and things for the next few weeks did improve.

On the way home one night from work, she called me, asked me to pull over, and then told me she was pregnant. "How far?" I asked, to which she replied 8 weeks. I was absolutely elated – all this time and finally we were there! I was going to be a Daddy at last.

When I returned home, expecting a huge hug and celebrations to be the order of the evening, I was somewhat shocked at the response. All she kept saying was, "What if ..." this and "What if ..." that; nothing but worries. "Wooo," I said, "all this isn't good for the baby – just calm down and we'll go through each of your worries one by one together, ok?" But this wasn't working – as calm as I was, she was going through the roof with anxiety and worry.

So I said we needed to see a doctor, but she was very reluctant, and I did think at the time that was a bit strange. She wouldn't come with me and insisted she would calm down as she sat there, and as I talked to her, she did seem to be a little steadier. Then she suggested that I should go and tell our neighbours the news (they had become good friends very quickly). I said I wasn't leaving her, and she told me not to be so possessive: "This isn't how it's going to be, is it? You can't be with me 24/7." I'm now pretty sure why she was behaving like this, but at the time, it wouldn't have occurred to me – it just all seemed odd. Anyway, reluctantly, I went round to the neighbours on my own and told them the good news.

But as with everything in my life (well, in my perception), this euphoria wasn't to last for too much longer. Very shortly after going to bed, she jumped out and rushed to the bathroom, screaming that she'd had a miscarriage. I was gutted. Just over ten years and now this! I was trying to be considerate and caring, but deep down, I was so angry. In my head, this was all her fault – all that worrying and stressing had caused this. I tried to keep those thoughts and feelings to myself and calmly said she needed to see a doctor. So that's what happened. We went to hospital, and they confirmed that it was a miscarriage brought on by stress (that didn't help me at all and just made my blood boil). When they said they wanted to keep her in overnight, that was a relief, to be honest.

What's clear to me now is that after telling me she really

wanted children she in fact never really wanted to have a baby and was deliberately trying to bring on a miscarriage. And it worked. I later discovered that all our married life, bar three months, she was on the contraceptive pill and had no intention of having any children. And what is even more painful is that my doctor – who was also hers – must have known all along, but because of the great British law of ethics, he could not say anything unless he wanted to lose his job. What a situation he was in – knowing that the husband really wanted children but also knowing the wife was doing her best not to conceive. The sad thing was that I did not want to be an old dad, and sadder than that is that I didn't want a baby with just anyone – I wanted to have a child with someone I loved and respected. But to have that decision taken from me without me even knowing angered me for a long time, and I think justifiably.

So here we were back to square one – still no baby. Not many weeks after this happened, I got a phone call from my sister that stunned me. Now, my sister hated children and never had any intention of ever having any. With all the boyfriends she'd had, any mention of children and they were out. But she had met someone who was the same as my father – very arrogant, selfish, two-faced, and pretentious (in my opinion), and a liar to boot. (I had actually found him out of a lie with my sister's assistance.) but she was absolutely besotted by him. And here she was on the phone saying that she had good news and that she was pregnant.

Well ... I did not know what to say. In those brief seconds that she told me, there must have been a hundred thoughts pinging round my head. My wife was standing next to me and had heard everything – she took the phone off me and talked to my sister – or rather, listened to my sister telling her all about it. Then after she put the phone down, my wife started on me, saying how rude I had been to my sister. I really couldn't believe I was hearing this. My wife expected me to congratulate my sister and thought I was rude for not doing this. I reminded her about what we had just lost only a few weeks ago and also the hatred that my sister had for children, but it was no good – she just thought I should have at least pretended that I was happy for her. Acting/pretending never was a strong point of mine (hence not being an actor!). I couldn't pretend, and why should I? I thought it was my sister who should be apologizing for being so insensitive and selfish.

***

Shortly after this happened (as if fate was trying to keep my mind occupied), my mother's mother passed away. (I wasn't as close to this Nanna because my father had made it quite difficult for me to see much of her). The day after the funeral, my mum's sister called me and said, "Can you come to your mum's as quick as you can? We have had to call the doctor out as your mum seems to be going crazy, shouting and screaming and crying uncontrollably."

I said, "I'll be there as soon as I can." A note here is that I was (as always) second choice to console my mother as, when they called my sister, she said she was too busy with customers working as a hair dresser. Within an hour, I was at the door of my mother's bungalow, and as I stepped in, my mother came flying out of the bedroom and flung her arms round my neck, saying, "James, thank God you're here!" This took me aback somewhat. In fact, as she had her arms round my neck, my own arms were outstretched straight behind her, and I actually had to instruct my own arms to hug my mother back. This was strange but not unexpected r – apart from when I was a baby, she never ever cuddled me, and in later years when I tackled her about this, she just said, "You weren't that kind of boy." To this day, I will never understand how you can justify not hugging your own child, but that was just how it was – all my hugs came from my Nanna.

***

Also around this time, something serious happened between my Nanna and me (on my dad's side). I lived some 25 miles away from her, but if I had work in Bury St Edmunds and I finished early for whatever reason, I would pop and see her. On this occasion, we were just sitting having a natter and a cup of tea when there was a bang on the door. I answered the door to save my Nanna's legs and there stood (well, just about still standing) my uncle's girlfriend covered in blood, all round her face and down her top. I was gobsmacked. I helped her (I'll call her Steph) into the kitchen and called my Nanna.

After a few minutes of cleaning up, I asked Steph, "What happened?" No sooner had these words come out of my mouth than my Nanna chipped in and said, "She's tripped over in the garden again – she's always doing it!"

"Is that what really happened?" I asked. "Have you been drinking?"

Suddenly she started to cry. She said "Sorry" to my Nanna but then told the truth – it was my uncle's doing, and it wasn't the first time.

I put my boots on and was just about to go out of the door when my Nanna got hold of my arm (I didn't know she could move that quick!) and asked me what I was doing. I replied, "If Phil (my uncle) wants to hit someone, well, I'm going to give him the chance – he can hit me!"

To my complete surprise, she said, "If you go round there and lay a hand on him, I'll never speak to you again." I knew that as the youngest he was always my Nanna's favourite, but he had been beating his girlfriend! I tried to defend my actions by saying, "Nanna how can you condone this behaviour? This is what your husband did to you, and that's why your father took you away from him. You have been in Steph's shoes. Now you're saying it's alright because it's Phil, your baby boy? Nanna, this isn't right." She wouldn't have it and just kept saying the same thing, that if I went near him, she'd never speak to me again.

This was *my* Nanna. I didn't want to fall out with her; she was the only person who'd listened to me and showed me any love when I was a child, and yet here I was arguing with her over her drunken, wife-beating waster of a son. Unfortunately, I said to her as I was leaving, "Nanna, I'm sorry, but this is just not right, and neither are you."

I did not speak with her for a number of weeks after that incident, but I did write to her explaining the trouble I was having with her decision to stand by her son over me. Unfortunately, we never spoke ever again. I've got a lot of regrets with my life, some brought on by me and many not, but not making peace with my Nanna is my number one to this day. I was being totally obstinate and not giving one inch, and by the same token neither was she, but I should have done something to pull it around. Principles, hey! Over the years they have cost me thousands of pounds and in this case cost me something that all the money in the world couldn't buy. My Nanna. So if there is an afterlife, I will just say, "I'm so sorry Nan," and hug the life out of her. If only.

***

In the meantime, I was working hard on the home. I got invited to price for a job for someone, and I agreed to do it even though it was in Southend.

Southend was well over 100 miles away from me, but whilst working there all week, I noticed that I didn't even miss my wife. In fact, to the contrary – I actually felt free and didn't even want to answer the phone when she would call me and ask if I was missing her. I certainly wasn't missing all the arguments, that was for sure, and that told me something critical, which really I had known for many years. It was time to call an end to this sham – because that was what it was. So upon finishing the contract and returning home, that was what I did. I called it a day on my thirteen-year marriage, and when I told her I wanted to split, she was not best pleased at all – the first thing she said was, "Why?"

With so many reasons in my head, underneath, I was boiling and really wanted to shout, "WHY? Where do I start? Where have you been for the past thirteen years?" But I really didn't want to get into yet another argument, so I said, "Let's sit down and work it out." Well, we started to, until she turned the waterworks on, but nothing was going to stop me this time (we had split up before a couple of times, but me being stupid, I came back). I also need to add at this point that I had reduced my tablets by half and in my mind was feeling the best I had for a long time and was hoping to build on this. Moving on from my acrimonious marriage seemed the right next step.

Without children, I thought this would be straightforward – pay off the mortgage and any other debts (especially any debts that I may not know of), then sell the home and split everything else money-wise 50/50. So I suggested that I take on the current house as it still needed a lot of work done and with the other half of the equity Elizabeth could buy a house near her mum and dad with a very small mortgage. If anything needed doing before moving in, I would come and do it for her – there wasn't any need to be horrible to each other, and if we could stay friends, I would always be there for jobs or anything in the future. With this said, she seemed to be more accepting of the situation that we were facing (both never having been through divorce before). Over the next couple of weeks, I would sort the mortgage situation out – in principle, the mortgage company would let me take it on and pay her off, so that's what I told her. Now, normally, she would argue over literally everything, however small or insignificant, and I was expecting her to say, "Well, you've got what you want now, haven't you, the whole house to yourself." I expected her not to want to split up at all. But when I told her this, she didn't argue or shout or have a go, which, although a pleasant change, did leave me with a bit of trepidation about what was happening.

Elizabeth then said she was going away for a few days to her cousin in Lincolnshire. I knew she indeed did have a cousin in Lincolnshire, so never thought any more about it. Three or four times she went off to her cousin, and I never read anything into this – I just thought it was her way of dealing with the breakup.

I had to go back to Southend to do some extras to the original works on the contract/construction job and Elizabeth was looking after Max. On the way home, I could see I was getting low on fuel. I always tried to go to the same supermarket filling station – I had got a loyalty card for Elizabeth, so every time I filled up with diesel, she would get all the points. They soon built up to a sizable amount that she would inevitably spend on herself. It was pretty ironic then that, when I was trying to be generous and still getting loyalty points for her, I saw what I was about to see …

So here I was, pulling into the supermarket car park before swinging round to the right to head for the filling station, when, as my van headlights swung round, I caught sight of what seemed to be the front of my car. As I slowed I thought, *That can't be my car*, because if Elizabeth was here shopping, she was so lazy she would have parked the car practically in the shop itself. But as I drew closer, I could see it was indeed my car, and I could also see the outline of my dog in the back seat. But what I couldn't see was any occupants – well, not at first. I wanted to know what was going on, so I pulled the van right opposite my car. Then as I was parked there, two heads popped up. One was Elizabeth (in the driver's seat) – now who was the other? It definitely was not her cousin, since the cousin in question was female and this clearly was a male. So that's what she had been doing at the weekend …

I sat there for a few minutes, then jumped out of my van and walked over to the passenger side of the car they were in – *my* car. I could see my wife doing up the buttons on her blouse … I didn't even give myself the chance to think about anything more. I just stopped at the door, then saw this man press the button to lock all the doors. Briefly, I thought, *Coward*, and told him to unlock the car. As his hand nervously pressed the button, I moved to the back door, got Max in my arms, and then took him back to my van. As I was returning to my driver's side, my wife was fully dressed and coming round the front of the van saying, "It's not what you think!" I thought, *Not what I think? No, course not.* I didn't answer her protestation of innocence – I just told her to get out of my way, and after the third time of telling, I just accelerated as she jumped away from the front of my van, and I sped off.

Ironically, I still had not filled up with fuel, and by the time I had realised, I was already ten miles away and nearly home. Upon getting home, I sent Elizabeth a text message to say I had put all her clothes outside in front of the skip. I told her to collect them before it was emptied on Monday or I would put all of them in the skip myself.

On the Sunday morning, she returned, and I helped load the car (our car) up with her clothes. Then she said there were things in the house that were hers, so I opened the front door and told her to help herself.

I had to say something. "How could you do this to me? I never ever strayed, even when we hadn't had sex for over a year. Never." She said nothing. Then I nearly made the worst mistake of my life (next to what had happened with my Nanna) and said to her, "You'll have to take Max. I have to work, and with a mortgage on my own, it'll have to be full time. I can't look after him the way he deserves – you'll have to look after him. Promise me." She just nodded, and I put all his things in the car with just enough space for him to sit. I shouted as she drove off, "Just look after him!" and returned into the house and sobbed and sobbed. But then I saw one of his toys left behind and realised I couldn't let him go. Thinking she wasn't ever going to let me have him back or she was going to use him against me, I phoned her and said (fighting back the tears), "Bring him back, *please* bring him back. He needs to be here." Well, to my surprise, she said, "OK," and within twenty minutes, she pulled up and I got him out of the car and just hugged him. Then I got his belongings and, still struggling with my tears, I said, "Thank you, I'll be in touch."

CHAPTER 17

And so to divorce

I didn't get a chance to get in touch with her because within a week I had a solicitor's letter. I wanted to keep it out of the solicitors, knowing from my first relationship break-up what a bunch of parasitic vultures they are, but it seemed it was out of my hands. (I must just add that in recent liaisons with my current solicitor, I now would say that they are definitely *not* all the same.)

Over the next few weeks, things got worse and worse. Elizabeth was now living with her new man, and I was on my own 24/7 with only Max to keep me company. I couldn't do anything to the house because she was wanting more and more money, and it looked like I would end up losing the house anyway. So I was just stuck there, and as much as I loved Max, he could not talk to me or listen, not like a human. Though in other ways, he was far better than a human, especially the one I was trying to divorce.

I was getting desperately lonely, and the feelings and negative thoughts were taking hold again. I could not rationalize the thoughts, and my mood was starting to slip quite rapidly. I had already increased the tablets but was now running out of them at speed, so I had to make an appointment with the local mental health team to get a review and also needed visits from the community psychiatric team again. At the first appointment, there were two nurses who asked me if I'd taken any action on the subject of suicide (or as I like to call it, self-termination; a lot less stigma to that term). I came clean and gave them the ten boxes of paracetamol that I had been collecting. I also had a bottle of vodka – if I drank it neat with the tablets, I reckoned it would make me so sick the tablets would not stay down long enough to poison my system, so I also had a special bottle of blackcurrant to mix just to make the process more bearable. The CPNs said I could keep the vodka, but I didn't drink alcohol anyway so I let them take that too.

I can remember sitting on the floor with Max and wishing to God that I hadn't asked for the divorce, because having someone you argued with 80% of the time was better than being lonely. I was struggling with my mindset – the will of my mind wanted desperately to get me firmly back to that 'safe place' and shut down into depression. I feel I have two main minds and not one. One wants so desperately to get on and do things, whilst the other, nearly as desperately, wants to give in to the 'security' of the depressive side. I seem to be trapped in the middle of these two minds – how frustrating is that?

Struggling on, not working much, and visiting my solicitor at least once a week, I had got to know the paralegal quite well. I was trying desperately to hide any depressive feelings and being jovial as much as I could. I sensed that this woman had feelings for me, just from a couple of things she said, and even though I hadn't any intentions of starting something whilst still being trapped in the past relationship, it was quite reassuring that someone else was interested in me.

But just after a year of trying to sort out finances, I was stunned when my wife filed for a divorce on the grounds of 'unreasonable behaviour'. This news just knocked me for six. In fact, I was so disgusted with this that I took the paperwork and drove to her parents' work place. Her father was sitting drinking a cup of tea (as he was always), and I threw this paperwork on the bench just as my nearly ex mother-in-law came out of the office to see what was going on. As they looked at me, I just couldn't control my emotions and started crying, but this was mixed with anger, and I shouted at them, "Read it!" Then whilst I could still speak, I said, "I hope you're both proud of what you've brought up; that's the sort of daughter you've got!" And with that, I snatched the paperwork back and walked out. They called out to me to stay and talk, but I just kept walking.

The next day, things got even worse. I visited my solicitor and sat at the huge table in the main front room of this lovely Georgian building, waiting for the paralegal to see me. When she came through the door and sat down, I noticed immediately things had changed – she was much more formal. I said to her, "How can this be right? Please tell me her solicitor has got this wrong." But she hadn't got it wrong. You see, in this country,(UK) someone can apply for a divorce on the grounds of unreasonable behaviour, and even an *illness*, through no fault of your own, can be classed as unreasonable behaviour. Isn't this ridiculous and sickening? And because this was filed by her first, there wasn't a thing I could do about it.

But getting to my other point: the paralegal who had definitely been interested in me suddenly wasn't interested at all after finding out what the 'unreasonable behaviour' was. In my experience, that's what can happen – when a woman finds out that a man she is interested in has had mind difficulties, often she will run for the hills. Don't get me wrong, I'm sure there may be some exceptions out there, but it seems to me that unless you are rich or famous or both, it's best if you keep your mental health situation to yourself. Which in itself can be very frustrating and debilitating. But is it worth the risk? Well, that decision would be yours.

At this point, I was seething and struggling to stay buoyant. I got home with my mind racing. I'd had enough of this whole situation with my wife shafting me, thanks to the laws in this country. I really was sick of the whole lot. So whilst walking Max, I thought of a way of ending everything, and I meant *everything*. I thought, *Why should I terminate my life for the sake of other people who are not worthy of being alive, the way they are treating me?* So I went to my local garage and filled two cans with petrol decanted them into other containers, and did this a few times until I had quite a few gallons of neat petrol in the back of my van. Then I went to where Elizabeth was living with her new man (which I found out by following him home one night) and parked on the other side of the road. I just sat there knowing what was going through my mind …

Suddenly, Max – my best friend by now – sat up and moved to the middle seat, sitting bolt upright and looking straight at the house, or so I thought, until he looked back at me and then licked me. I couldn't get the thoughts out of my head: the thought that not only would I take these two parasites out, I'd be finished too – no more depression, no more desperation, peace at last. I was so tired from the past, and these thoughts were getting stronger and stronger. With a lighter in my hand and tears again rolling down my cheeks, I kissed my boy and said, "Sorry, mate." For some reason, he then started barking, and he had a bloody good bark. I was panicked then, and I didn't as a rule get panicked. But I did suffer from embarrassment and hated being looked at, especially in a crowd. And here we were in a van with enough petrol in the back to blow up half the street if it hit a gas main – and that was my aim, to hit the gas box on the front of the house. But I couldn't stop Max from barking, and passers-by were now looking over to the van. I had to get out of here, and so, as the engine was already running, all I had to do was accelerate, and we were off.

I drove through the town and he was still barking. and this was unusual behaviour for him because, apart from when instructed or excited, he hardly ever barked. It wasn't until we were about three miles away that he stopped, and I pulled over. I said to him, "What was all that about, Max?" and he just looked at me and barked again, but only the once. I returned home, spoke to my neighbour, who was now a good friend, and told him what had happened. As he was a gardener, he agreed to take the petrol off my hands to use in the mower. You can draw your own conclusions, but Max behaving like that felt like intervention to me.

So we were divorced (ironically, the day before our wedding anniversary), and within a month of this, Elizabeth was re-married to the man that had had his hands firmly in my pockets for the past year and was draining me faster than a Ferrari doing 0–60. After 18 months of instability, going back and forth to court and not knowing whether I was going to have any money left, we had the final court appearance. My now ex-wife could not even look at me, and her new husband had left her to face me alone and was in the pub opposite the courthouse. But the situation was finally at an end.

By now, I was 'maxed out' on the anti-depressants but still standing (only just though), and it was time to look at what mess I was in. Because you just get swept along with the whole scenario and just want it to end. Well, let's see where I was. I was mortgaged to the hilt, my business overdraft was way beyond its max, and then my bank foreclosed on me, and I had to finish renovating a house that was only just habitable. So I went to work on the house using credit cards, just trying to pay the bills and finish renovating the whole house to a top standard. But the housing market was dropping so fast that once the house was completed, if I had sold then, I would have been lucky to get £15,000 out of it, and what the heck was I supposed to do with that amount? After twenty years working, that's all I would end up with, so I had no choice – I would have to rent it out. When I instructed the local letting agents I was maxed out on all my credit cards and owing nearly £30k. I had nothing at all apart from £3 in my pocket.

When the sign went up, a neighbour came and knocked on my door and said her daughter needed somewhere to live. So, long story short, I rented it to her. But she couldn't move in for two weeks, so I wouldn't get the deposit and the first month's rent till then. I was a bit stuck, and I wasn't about to ask my mother for any money (a pride thing, I guess), but on the other hand, I couldn't last two weeks on £3. So I gathered up all the scrap I had lying down the side of the house and took it the scrap man. I thought, *If I only get 60 quid for this, we can live off that for two weeks,* but as it was, he gave me £320 for it. I couldn't believe it – I could have kissed him. So I didn't have to ask my mother for money, but I did accept her offer to stay in her box room with Max, just for a while!

Over the next few months, I was juggling a number of credit cards plus loans and still trying to pay each one down a bit and, of course, still live. Even my accountant said to me one day, "James , I don't know how you are going to get out of this financial mess – have you looked into declaring yourself bankrupt?" I said I didn't want to go down that route if at all possible, due to the fact that I believed I would have a black mark against me for the rest of my days, no matter what the law said. He replied, "I totally understand, but honestly – I can't see how you are going to manage *not* going down that route. It was a testing time. I was still seeing the CPN on a fortnightly basis and seeing a psychologist once a month, keeping my contact with them open, which was important.

CHAPTER 18

Freedom and changes

Even though I was heavily in debt and on my own, to me, this time was like a breath of fresh air. I obviously felt still angered and frustrated, but I was free. Free from my now ex-wife and the constant arguing, free to do things that I wanted to do but she never would.

One change I noticed after the divorce came through was an improvement in my physical health. I had been diagnosed with severe IBS (irritable bowel syndrome) to the point of not being able to stand up straight in the morning, the pain was so bad. I eliminated a huge number of foods from my diet to try to reduce the frequency and severity of the pain, but it still remained. The doctors said if it wasn't the diet, then it was my work stress, through being self-employed. But as soon as I was divorced, suddenly it went. (In the 13 years since then, I haven't had any symptoms at all and I eat whatever I like, including hot curries, which were definitely off the menu when married.) I also used to suffer from at least 3–4 migraines a month that were so severe they would knock me out for two days at a time, and now I probably only get five a year.

Another change was weight loss. You see, because I had been bouncing from times of just misery to deep clinical depression, I really was, 90% of the time, unhappy with most things. So I used to comfort eat. I knew from my previous years when training in the gym that what I was eating wasn't doing me any good, but it felt like I had nothing else to placate me. Even when I was doing manual work, the calorific intake of the rubbish I was eating was so high, the pounds just piled on, and before long, I was looking at being nearly 6 stones overweight – clinically obese. This was totally down to unhappiness and nothing else. But with the divorce, the weight started to go down. I had more control over what I was eating, and after the initial wobbly start of life on my own, I was eating far better. I was used to everyday stresses, having been self-employed for over 20 years by then, so overeating was without a doubt caused by the emotional stress.

Within the first three years of being on my own, I had got my weight back to the point where it should have been and have never put that amount of weight back on again.

As for my mental health … After the divorce, I also began to have more control over my thoughts. But this wasn't achieved overnight – it took time, but it can be done, as I've proved. Over-thinking can cause so many problems, but it can be challenged with CBT and/or psychotherapy. (Although on two occasions I had to refuse the CBT because I simply could not connect with the therapist – the right person will make a huge difference.)

I took antidepressants and later on SSRIs on and off for 24 years, but since 2010, I have not taken them at all. I do feel in more control of my mind than I ever did, and I think a huge factor is choosing who to be with in my life. Please ... I know it may be hard to do, but look at the person you are with and be honest with yourself. It would not be true to say that my ex-wife was all the cause of my recurring depression. But a psychiatrist once said to me when I was describing my relationship with her, "We would call someone like her a 'passive bully'." This means that anything I suggested or wanted to do, she would find ways to be negative about. After years of this, you start to question yourself. Her own mother had been on antidepressants for over 25 years of *her* marriage. So I think the message is if someone is making you ill (and in my wife's case, I really don't think it was on purpose – it was her character, either inherited or what she grew up with), then, as hard as it may be, you need to move on – life's too short, as they say. I went through a horrendous divorce, and in all it cost me a huge amount of money and mental torture, but to feel how I feel now ... it was worth every penny and every tear, every ache, and every pain to be free.

There have been changes, too – not all I have had control over, to be fair, but I think they are relevant and have complemented the conscious changes that I have made.

For example, as a child, I can't remember crying a great deal at all, and even into adulthood I don't have a huge recollection of crying, even at events that would require a tear or two. Like when the family dog died – the same dog that I walked all the time and spent a huge amount of time with – no tears. Splitting from loved ones – still no tears. But it wasn't because I didn't feel anything. I think it was a by-product of my upbringing where I hardly ever saw any tears, apart from my sister's from time to time. And because I was treated like an army recruit, crying seemed to be wimpy to me and something that I should not do. I thought I should be tough like a robot and not show any feeling. That was how I felt I was meant to behave.

But now, at nearly fifty years old, I can cry at the drop of a hat. I feel emotional at nearly everything, and it does take quite a lot of self-restraint to keep the tears back sometimes when I think it is inappropriate. This feeling, behaviour, or emotion all started when I divorced and decided to make changes to myself, personality-wise. I might not have been trying to show more emotion, but that happened as a sort of side effect of those changes. Being more affectionate is something I have had to consciously work on, and now it is as if I was always like that.

Another personality trait was worrying all the time. (I got that from my mother, who to this day is a compulsive worrier). But I have gone from being a worrier to not really worrying about anything at all. I think when you hit the bottom of life (*i.e.*, self-termination), really everything else pales into insignificance. Now I see things that I would have worried about as just a bit of aggravation and an inconvenience.

***

Now that I was on my own and occasionally had a bit of spare cash, which in the beginning was not often, I would buy books on anything to do with thinking, emotions, psychology, mindfulness ... in fact, anything associated with the mind, trying to have a better understanding. I had no idea how I would cope at this time with emotions and feelings of hate and resentment, but as I read more and more, I was starting to get an understanding of how my mind was working, and this could only be a good thing.

And it was. I finally managed to get to grips with the reincarnation theory and accepted this as something I could not control.

Everyone has a belief that will help them through the winding path of life. Whether it's religious or not is not really important, but we all have some belief or philosophy about life, even if we can't put it into words easily. Well, my beliefs changed, as you have already read, when I made a flippant remark to an uncle of mine and I read a book about reincarnation.

Unfortunately, at the time, I was definitely not in the right frame of mind to take the information that I had read, no matter how convincing it was to me. And I was definitely not willing then to accept the meaning of it. I think all my life I'd had self-control and a desire to control what was around me, especially situations which now I realise I actually had no control over at all. All this would do was create frustration and in turn anger and resentment. But I learnt that if I accepted what I couldn't alter and change, what was not in my control, then I could have a better existence than before.

I reasoned with myself that what I believed in, which I call *fate,* was my answer. I had to accept that my previous incarnation had indeed been of bad spirit and their conduct was obviously of the wrong kind. That believed, I then had to accept this situation and find a way of living with it.

Before I continue, I must stress that this is *my* belief, and, rightly or wrongly, it works for me. Many people, especially (in my experience) psychologists, don't believe in any form of religion or spiritualization, but funnily enough, many use the term *luck* and evidently believe in this. (I remember a specific psychologist saying: "That's just bad luck.")

Whether you call it *fate* (as I do) or any other name, be it God or Allah or even luck, to me, it does not matter, if it works for you. So I believe, in this *fate,* that I have a debt to pay, and some aspects of my life are a persecution or punishment for a previous existence. There are a lot of things that I have no control over whatsoever, and this is one of them – 'what will be will be'! That may seem a negative way to look at it, but once the acceptance had set in that this is how it is, it gave me a sense of calm from the frustrating anger that was driving me before.

In fact, for a number of years, it has given me a sense of immortality. The fact is, I believe that my 'sentence' must be long-term and for me to be cut down (so to speak) before the end of the journey wouldn't make sense. I do realise that the journey/persecution will come to an end, but I don't know when that will be any more than anyone else. But for the time being, I really believe it will be for a number of years yet. So although I have a number of non-life-threatening ailments, which are really a daily annoyance, if I didn't have this belief, I could quickly become much more angry or depressed. Accepting that these things are part of my life for a reason helps me to cope with them better. For me, it's all down to *fate* – I had to find a way to work with it instead of fighting against it, because that's a fight I can never win.

Some things I've seen on the news really confirm this belief of fate to me. For example, an aeroplane with 250 people on board crashes and only 10 survive. Why? Why did those 10 survive and the other 240 all die? Why were the survivors from all parts of the plane? To me, the answer is *fate,* or, as some would say, "their time wasn't up."

A man runs along a beach with a semi-automatic gun, firing indiscriminately at no given target – as he creates havoc across the beach, some people get shot and others don't, even though they are all lying down on the sand. Why? In this particular scenario, that happened in Tunisia. Ine man lay on top of his wife to protect her, only for his wife to be shot, but he didn't get hit. How was this?

In the past, I have worked my backside off in an attempt to

create a business, and for whatever reason, it has just not been successful. If I had done everything I could to make it work, then again, why? Some singer/songwriters find a recording contract nearly instantly and others of the same calibre seem to go on for years knocking on doors and gigging without a big break – again, why? If you have heard the saying "You have to be in the right place at the right time," oh, how true that is. I call this *fate*; others call it luck or destiny. Paul McCartney has said on many occasions when interviewed that he has been very lucky with his career – and obviously thought that talent and skill were important, but without a smattering of 'lady luck', well, need I say more? Apart from personally I think he is one of the most talented music artists there is.

So the belief that I finally did accept is now nowhere near the burden it was. From time to time it's still frustrating but it doesn't lead my thoughts to such dark places anymore.

I have had to learn to understand my attitude towards principles and hypocrisy. Many would believe these are learnt behaviours and certainly not inherited, but in my experience, it does not seem to be true. I have said previously in the book that I am a principled person, but I don't believe I am like this because of what I learnt from my parents. My mother was just submissive, and my father would tell me that he was very principled but his actions would not show this. However, I do have an uncle on my father's side who would stand by his principles at any cost. I think this has been passed on to me genetically, and for once, this is a trait from his side that I am content to have. But it still needs to be kept in perspective, otherwise it could lead down the wrong road, especially if you have a tendency to be a little obsessive about them (principles, that is).

I have trouble tolerating hypocrisy, as I saw it constantly from my father. This *definitely* is behaviour that, as a child, I observed from the adults around me. As with everything in life, there are grey areas where what you do or say could be construed as hypocrisy, such as not telling the full truth to save someone from unnecessary hurt. I think it's the blatant hypocrisy that I would see that I have trouble with. Some of the time, this behaviour would be mixed with the old adage of "You will do as I say and not as I do." Each time I 'put my head above the parapet', I find myself questioning whether I'm being true to myself or being a hypocrite.

Another behaviour I think is really important to mention is perfectionism. This one did nearly kill me (literally) as it was something I had drilled into me – "Near enough is not good enough." That was irony if ever there was, coming from my father, who, as it turned out, was the least perfect person I knew.

But having this constantly drummed into me from a very early age really did cause me huge problems in adulthood. I had great difficulty realising and accepting that there was no such thing as perfection. I wasted so much time beating myself up because things I had done were not perfect – could I have done better? Is 95% enough? Why didn't I get 100%? I put in 100% effort, so why only 95%? At one point, this was torture to my self-worth, not to mention my mind's health. With my work in the construction industry, I would constantly strive to achieve perfection in the running of my business, both in the level of workmanship from myself but also from others who worked for me. You can see the way this would end – yes, with me crashing into an angry and then depressive state and the business closing.

This desire for perfection would cause me to argue intensely with others, which was totally unfair, but it was entrenched in me. It was my father who made me believe that perfection was the only way. And what he said went, like it or not.

He would go through fads of interests or hobbies. One time when he was building a fishpond and asked me to help, I asked about the design. (I was and still am very interested in the design element) Because the patio at the rear of the house was square, he said to me, "In design, if what's around you has a square theme, then you definitely don't mix in curves and circles. It has to have straight lines."

I used to be completely submissive to my father. Unfortunately, this meant I really did believe everything he told me as factual – who wants to think that their father isn't Superman or Einstein? It wasn't until I started investigating these facts later in my life that I came to the realisation that he was just making things up on subjects that he really didn't know about to keep up the pretence of knowing it all. Because of his opinionated arrogance, what he said did, for many, many years, dictate my own opinion. It took many years of torment before I started to understand through psychological therapy that all I was doing was holding myself back from a life. Unfortunately, after having had those opinions forced onto me for so long, it was incredibly hard to move on in life, not knowing what to believe in your own head.

Design, as it turns out, is something I love and genuinely feel very passionate about, which has led me to looking at many different periods of architecture and design for many things, from tea sets to cars, from furniture to houses – so I wonder, for instance, if you shouldn't combine circles with squares, did the art deco period have it all wrong?

Because you are told by your parents or loved ones that something is meant to be that way, it doesn't necessarily mean it's a fact. It's worth investigating further and finding out for yourself. On the other hand, you may have genuine parents who would be totally honest with you if they didn't really know an answer. *Wow*, what a father that would be –and I know they are out there.

I believe this insistence on being right stems from arrogance – very strong on my father's side. About eight years ago, I was having a conversation with my mother when she said probably the most offensive thing (to me, that is): "You sound just like your father!" Well, this really cut deep, and since then, I have kept on improving my manner and curtailing any attitude of arrogance that I can detect, which is quite draining itself, but it can be done.

Just recently, I found myself apologising to a friend if the last time we met I came over as a bit arrogant. He replied, "What arrogance?" I don't think he will ever know what a compliment he had given me, and it is also proof that the changes that I have made and continue to make to be a better person are working.

You can indeed change your personality if you want to, need to, or feel you should. You can also pick parts of others' personalities that you may like or respect and start using those in with yours, and after a while these will become part of you.

I am very conscious all the time of my personality and keep monitoring it whilst trying to improve it. In the beginning, it was quite draining, but now it is a lot easier to manage, and I am finally becoming the person I want to be– a person who I can respect instead of resent and even loathe at certain times. These changes have all been achieved by therapy from the last ten years – self-therapy and an awful lot of reading   .

***

I need to explain the terms '**forgiveness**' and '**acceptance**' just in case it seems a bit strange or is misinterpreted.

First, **Forgiveness:** this term applies mainly to oneself, to take what you have started with, whether it is behavioural, spiritual, social, or biological, and learn to work with it instead of against it. We are all born with a certain physical makeup, and if you just lived with what you were born with, then the likes of Arnold Schwarzenegger would never have achieved any of the many accolades as a champion bodybuilder for the simple reason that a person with, say, a naturally thick waist (genetically speaking) could not change this part of their antimony, so they would work with what they have and alter other parts of their body to give the impression that the waist was smaller (i.e., build the shoulder mass up), then ascetically they would seem to have a much smaller waist. You need to forgive yourself (or Mother Nature in this case) for your beginnings and work with it.

The same goes for the mind, although some believe that we are born with a clear mind, ready to accept instructions, while others believe that we already have preconceived notions and ideas in our brains. Either way, right from our earliest memories, we absorb information like a sponge, and unfortunately, our parents or overseers will, often, be the cause of what we have to forgive. Yet again forgiveness that is required and also whatever you have inherited in the ways of traits (good or bad).

Whatever behaviours you have been accustomed to can be changed, even parts of your personality that you do not like or find hard to accept. Again, there is a BUT, and that is, it's not easy to undertake, and although it requires a huge amount of work and commitment, it can be done. I have done this, and now instead of living an existence, I'm living a life. Now that has to be worth all the hard work, wouldn't you agree?

Secondly, **Acceptance:** now this was and is to this day a big one for me. One that I will probably (no! definitely) struggle with for the rest of my life, BUT because of acceptance, at least I have a life, whereas before, constantly going from one episode of my mind's trauma to another year in year out wasn't a life at all. It was just an existence that at some point I would have terminated had I not found a way of accepting the things I couldn't do anything about. In my case, it was new (non-religious) beliefs that helped with this.

Yet again, the word 'belief' can be challenged as something they may appear true to you but not to others. Personally, it doesn't really matter to me whether my beliefs are factually correct or not –as long as it works for the person in question and the beliefs do not have a detrimental effect on your behaviour to the point of hurting others, which mine do not at all.

All round the world, there are societies built on beliefs of all different kinds, not just religious, and unfortunately, some of the people who have beliefs do, from time to time, let them get out of hand, and the result is hurting others.

My beliefs actually saved my life and gave me the freedom to actually have some sort of life – it all comes down to acceptance. There is nothing I can do to change what is, so I learnt to accept it and live with it. As the saying goes que sera sera – whatever will be, will be!

CHAPTER 19

Final thoughts

Unfortunately, all these behaviours seen as children, whether we learn to be the same or not, do have a massive effect on our adult lives. For some, like me, they do need to be addressed before we cause ourselves and others unintentional hurt and suffering.

To this day, I have moments when the words, *Is this the best I can do?* still rattle in my mind, and I have to consciously get a grip of those feelings and thoughts before they escalate. But again, this is behaviour and a way of thinking that, even though entrenched from a childhood of bullying, has been addressed, and now does not dominate my life nearly so much as it once did.

When people ask, "were they born like that or was it his/her environment?" well, what a question. Our minds control us completely – we are our mind, but what is around us bombards us (or it filters through, as with passive bullying). Either way, this has a huge effect on our actions, reactions, responses, decisions ... in fact, everything we do and say. If you see a psychologist, they will say, "Let's start with your childhood." And my childhood experiences must have had a huge influence on my health, as well as some of my decisions and choices. *I do not think parents fully realise, when holding their new addition to their family, what a responsibility they have taken on and what an impact they will have on the child.* Obviously, what you inherit from your parents you do not have any control over, to a degree. You need to understand what sort of person *you* are, to give yourself the best advantage to cope or get on with your life.

I was once diagnosed as having a 'personality disorder', having been born from two opposing personality types, and instead of having (as my sister has) a strong bias to one parent or the other (in her case, she is just like my father), I had more of a 60/40 mix, which caused a lot of confusion and anger. Until I started to fully understand what parts were what, I really was struggling. So I guess my message in relation to this is to not be too hard on yourself. Just try to look deep inside and do your best to understand and, if necessary, forgive yourself; find some equilibrium that you can live with.

The same goes for the mind – you can change this, even parts of your personality that you do not like or find hard to accept. It's not an easy task to undertake, but although it is a lot of hard work and commitment, it has worked for me, and I am now living a *life* instead of living an *existence*. Now, that has to be worth all the hard work, hasn't it?

I also think it's time to tackle the stigma of such problems and the negatives associated with the term 'mental health'. I would love to see one day a whole revolution of change with the behaviour, the prejudice, the stigmas, and total lack of understanding and care of the *mind's health*, because it seems like the majority of the general public look at the term 'mental health' as something to be totally ashamed of. But it is just an illness of the mind – it doesn't make you a worse person to deal with or to talk to or to do business with. In fact, the term 'mental health' in itself is the same as the term 'diet' that everyone associates with restriction or forbidden foods. Every person on the planet is on a diet already, be it a diet of pizza, chips, burgers, etc., or a diet of low fat foods. So the term in the way people perceive it is actually incorrect, and the meaning is incorrect as well. The same goes for the term 'mental health' - we all have our own mental health going on all the time in our minds. It's just that sometimes, as with the body, it falls ill or needs to be repaired. But unlike the body, you can't see the damage or defected part to correct, unlike a broken arm or leg. Unfortunately, the mind is not so easily accessible, and for 90% of us, to see a picture of our brain when not working correctly (if it could be seen), we would not understand what we were looking at.

And the problem isn't going to go away on its own. Nowadays, with the internet, the bullying (the cause of many of my problems) has carried on through technology. (I am now confident that if I had a son or daughter who was being bullied as I was, I would be able to give positive advice to combat this and enable them to move forward. I only wish there had been someone there for me at that time with some coping mechanisms or good advice.)

I would not tell any of my customers that I had an illness of the mind. People (i.e., celebrities) who have plenty of money can afford to take time off to gather their thoughts or have therapy without the worry of not paying the mortgage, but for the less fortunate (particularly the self-employed), this is a totally different story that really needs addressing. I have been there many times, and it does nothing for your recovery when the wolf is knocking down the door, I can tell you. When mental health organisations say that opinions are changing ... well, I don't know where they are getting their information from, but in my experiences, opinion is not changing much, and if it is, it is definitely not quickly enough. The stigma is still very prevalent and out there every day.

Also, on the subject of anti-depressants or SSRIs –I totally agree with the need to take them, whether for emotional support or for people who have low levels of serotonin in their brain. More people could have better mind health if they accepted that, for whatever reason, their body doesn't make sufficient amounts of serotonin for them to function properly and so they need to take a form of anti-depressants to address this situation. But so many people (especially men) feel that if they have to rely on a tablet to function more normally, it is a sign of weakness or even a disability. But is this any different from a person injecting themselves with insulin because their body doesn't produce enough of it? If they could see it as exactly the same scenario (which basically it is!), then I'm sure a small but significant amount of people would benefit immensely.

In wider society, it is often frowned upon to take tablets like antidepressants, yet it is cool amongst a number of people to take tablets for recreation. What a strange people we are!

I have proven that anyone can get on top of depression/ mental illness or learn to work/live with it. I realised that the thoughts, beliefs, perceptions … all could be challenged. If not challenged, I would get so mixed up with them that my mind would trigger a depressive episode to shut things down for a while. Eventually, I understood that this was 'self-preservation' – the pragmatic part of my brain would shut my mind down to save me from taking any form of action. The depression was like a safety valve to stop me from metaphorically exploding or destroying, or worse still, committing self-termination.

Which leads me to the state of desperation someone must be in to take his or her own life. The human body was made to survive at incredible costs (for example, drug users who are putting chemicals in their bodies on a daily basis and can keep doing this for decades and still have their body keep on going). To stop this fantastic piece of biology from surviving not only takes a huge amount of desperation but determination too, and guts, if I'm being brutally honest. To bring the human body to a stop takes a lot of fighting. In my case, it was fuelled by frustration and anger rather than depression.

It's still not fair or right to judge someone who has ended their life or tried to. The desperation they were suffering would have been immense. We need to be more understanding and tolerant of others who are suffering, and they *are* suffering – believe me, I know. Unfortunately, the other problem is the fact that a number of people use the terms 'depression' , 'anxiety issues', 'bi-polar disorder', and so on, as a reason not to work and instead claim from the tax payer (sorry, I mean government/state). All this will do is make a mockery of the genuine sufferers out there who really need help, and it will hinder the acceptance that your mental health is so important to keep healthy and in check (just as it is for your body).

***

I'm sorry if what I've written about in the 'final thought' chapter seems pretty bleak, but I'm afraid we are our own worst enemies, and until attitudes change about people's mind health, we really are going to struggle as a society. The numbers of people who are having to take time off work because of this is increasing year on year at an alarming rate – we as a society need to act now and embrace the situation. This isn't meant to sound like a rant or a soapbox speech, but it is something I am passionate about.

With a lot of commitment and acceptance, you can take some sort of control of your mind's health (or mental health, if you must) and live a more purposeful life with a lot more enjoyment than you would have thought possible. But it's not easy and it takes constant work, a bit like a computer that needs updates – that's how the mind works. Every now and then, it needs to rest and be cleared, ready for its new instructions/

updates. I do frequently monitor my mind's health and my behaviour – a constant maintenance programme, if you like! – so as not to be anything like the person I despise (my father). You will by now have made judgements about me from reading this book, but I would just like to say that had my father admitted at any point that he himself had problems that really needed addressing, and shown any remorse or understanding, I would not be so vehement about my opinion of him. I hope my father is in a minority and that most will have loving, caring, and honest parents. Enjoy, because not all will be like that, and you are the truly lucky ones.

Before this last page appears, and due to the fact that most of previous pages may have seemed more bleak than positive, I just wanted to share a short story with you on the subject of 'hope'. *(Be warned, that this story maybe triggering to survivors of sexual abuse)* This is something that, when entrenched in a battle with your own mind's health (mental health), can seem very hard to reach and hold on to. Hopefully, this story will help you as it did for me.

A young girl of 12 years in (shall we say) the far-east was sold by her family for money to buy food for her other six siblings. She was sold to the local town's police chief a long way from her village she had lived in. For the next two years, she carried out tasks for the chief and his wife/family (I suppose more as a slave than a nanny/home helper), doing all the chores that nobody else wanted to do, but at the age of fourteen, she was suddenly seen as a female who could do a lot more, and she was then being used as a sex object by the chief. Then on some nights, he would have some male friends round (and all drinking), and they would share his new toy (for a better way of describing her). She would be passed from one man to another without any say in the matter and abused in the most graphic ways. This went on until she was sixteen. One evening (as before), a number of the chief's (so-called) male friends come round, and as the evening progressed and the girl was, again being brutally abused, she found herself near the desk in the room where this was taking place and could see a gun laying in an open draw. The girl knew she could reach this gun, and, assuming it was loaded, she could have stopped this brutality, either killing her abuser/s or turning the gun on herself. I think most of us wouldn't have thought twice about stopping this abuse, one way or the other. But the girl didn't act on this situation, and instead she did what she had always done, wiping away the tears and putting a brave front on, as the chief didn't like the girl crying. You are probably thinking the same as I was: *What was she thinking? Why didn't she take the chance to end this?* Surely being in prison or dead would have been better than being sexually abused week in week out and treated like a piece of meat! About a month after her sixteenth birthday, there was a raid on the police chief's home, and he and a number of his so-called friends were all arrested for what had been happening over the past four years, and the girl was taken to a local nunnery for a time of recovery (not that anyone would ever fully recover from this sickening behaviour).

When with the nuns, she was asked why she hadn't acted on the circumstances with the gun. She said, "I had **hope** that one day somewhere, somehow, I would be rescued and saved, and that's what I truly believed." The hope was what kept her from death or causing a massacre, and she believed that a life in prison in her country would have been no better than what she was enduring. And as for death, with her hope of rescue, that wasn't an option for her.

I still find it hard to even imagine what she had been through and how much she must of hated her 'owner' Not sure I could have been through that and not defended myself – in fact, I know I couldn't have. Again, as I've said, it can be very difficult to see and feel hope when swamped with thoughts that are driving emotions in a very dark place.

Whatever your upbringing has been, you can change to be the person you want to be. But I would just say, look closely at yourself and your childhood – if you can say that you had parents who showed you unconditional love and tenderness, gave you praise (when praise was due/needed), supported and tried to understand you (irrelevant of their own thoughts/feelings), listened and gave you positive feedback on any given situation, but most importantly made you feel that you were loved and well thought of and worthy of being a person in your own right, only then you can be fully relaxed that your childhood will not have had an adverse effect on the life ahead of you. Nobody is perfect, but if you had parents who tried their best to be like that, you should be really grateful for them.

I know a lot of people will read this and think that you shouldn't blame your parents for your losses in life, but the facts speak for themselves – some legitimately have good reason to expect their parents to take some of the blame for their life as an adult. Whatever you feel about what I have written, those formative years *really* matter and will affect the rest of your life. Trust me – I know.

I had been in and out of clinical depression for over 20 years, but I finally did find a way to alter and cope with the things that I previously could not. It *can* be done, it *has* been done, and *you* can do it too.

Many people (including psychologists) have told me to find a way for forgiveness to enter my being. I have over the years battled with myself to find a way of forgiving, but when it comes to my father, it just isn't possible.

You see, I feel he robbed me of my childhood and nearly ended my adulthood prematurely. I know it was definitely not *all* down to him, but there is a huge amount that was, and because of that, I will never be able to forgive, and because I can't forgive, I will have to carry this stone around with me for the rest of my days. And if that were not bad enough, I have him haunt me every time I catch a glimpse of myself in the mirror.

Unless I grow a beard to cover 50% of my face (which I have done on a number of occasions), I am stuck with this torment and constant reminder of my past.

I understand when they say you need to let go and move on, but as many of you out there will know that sometimes it's just not that simple! Getting to grips with my mind's health was challenging enough, but achievable, but as for forgiveness, well, that one I will have to endure. I don't think now, looking back (especially after writing this book), the past is dictating to me in any way, so onwards!

My advice would be: change what you can change, *if* you should so wish. What you cannot change (fate) you need to accept and learn to live with! (I know this is sometimes easier said than done). If you go for a job or buy a house and it doesn't work out, then you weren't meant to have the house or the job. Unfortunately, you will probably never know why (that is the frustrating part, I admit). But that is the way it is; that's fate. You will, however, later on down the road, look back and start to surmise why you did not get that house or job. Now some will say that is a total waste of time, just move on! It's irrelevant, its history! All true, but, for some like myself, it helps with the moving forward process. If I have some idea/explanation of what happened in the past, I try to learn from what had happened, so as not to veer down that same path again. There is a reason for everything! But unfortunately, the reasons are not always very clear. But still there was a reason.

And my last words (for now) would be: wouldn't it be good to have a national Mind's Health Day and finally try to eradicate that terminology 'mental health'?

www.ingramcontent.com/pod-product-compliance
Lightning Source LLC
Chambersburg PA
CBHW062052270326
41931CB00013B/3038